Atlas of Gastrointestinal and Hepatobiliary Infections

An **Essential Slide Collection of Gastrointestinal
and Hepatobiliary Infections**, based on the
material in this book, is available. The collection
consists of numbered 35mm slides of each
illustration in the book, and each section is
accompanied by a slide index for easy reference.
The material is presented in an attractive binder,
which also contains a copy of the Atlas. The
essential slide collection is available from:

Gower Medical Publishing, Middlesex House
34–42 Cleveland Street, London W1P 5FB

Gower Medical Publishing
101 5th Avenue, New York, NY 10003, USA

Atlas of Gastrointestinal and Hepatobiliary Infections

W. Edmund Farrar MD, FACP
Professor of Medicine and Microbiology
Medical University of South Carolina
Charleston, South Carolina, USA

Martin J. Wood FRCP
Consultant Physician
East Birmingham Hospital
Birmingham, UK

Gower Medical Publishing • London • New York

Distributed in the USA and Canada by:

Raven Press Ltd
1185 Avenue of the Americas
New York
New York 10036
USA

Distributed in the rest of the world by:

Gower Medical Publishing
Middlesex House
34–42 Cleveland Street
London W1P 5FB
UK

Cataloguing in Publication Data:

Catalogue records for this book are available from
the US Library of Congress and British Library.

ISBN 1–56375–5556

The material in this book is derived from *Infectious Diseases: Text and Color Atlas* by W. Edmund Farrar, Martin J. Wood, John A. Innes and Hugh Tubbs (Gower Medical Publishing 1991).

Text set in New Baskerville; captions set in Futura Book.
Illustrations originated in Hong Kong by Mandarin.
Text origination and page make-up by Bright Arts (Hong Kong).
Printed in Hong Kong.
Produced by Mandarin Offset (Hong Kong).

Project Manager: Stephen McGrath

Design: Ian Spick

Illustration: Ian Spick
Lee Smith

Index: Nina Boyd

Production: Susan Bishop

Publisher: Michele Campbell

Preface

Infections of the gastrointestinal tract and liver cause an enormous amount of human suffering around the world. Diarrhoeal disease due to various bacterial pathogens and viruses is responsible for hundreds of millions of episodes of illness and several million deaths each year. Approximately 10% of the world's population is infected with *Entamoeba histolytica*, and helminthic infections afflict well over a billion individuals. Infection with the hepatitis B virus is present in approximately 250 million individuals worldwide, and infections due to the hepatitis A virus and non-A, non-B viruses are also extremely common.

In this realm of medicine as in many others a good illustration can often greatly facilitate the understanding of a disease process, or even lead directly to an accurate diagnosis. In this book we have tried to take full advantage of the visual possibilities, and have included clinical photographs, pictures of gross pathology, light and electron micrographs of histopathologic changes and microorganisms, and imaging studies utilizing radiological and radionuclide techniques. We hope and believe it will be valuable not only for gastroenterologists but also for other clinical workers who encounter these infections in their work.

Acknowledgements

This collection of slides could not have been assembled without the generous collaboration of many friends and colleagues in various parts of the world. We wish to express here our appreciation to all of them; the sources of individual slides are given in the captions.

Large groups of slides or other special help (or both) were provided by the following individuals: Dr J Robert Cantey, Dr John T Cunningham, Dr Herbert L Dupont, Dr Christopher Edwards, Professor Alasdair M Geddes, Dr Gordon R Hennigar, Dr Thomas W Holbrook, Dr R Duren Johnson, Dr Stewart Knutton and Dr Jo Newman.

Finally, we thank Carver and Stephanie for their essential support and encouragement in this effort.

WEF
MJW

Charleston and Birmingham, 1992.

Contents

Chapter 1

Oesophageal and Gastric Infections

INFECTIOUS OESOPHAGITIS

The two most important aetiological agents in infectious oesophagitis are *Candida* species and the herpes simplex virus. Both of these infections are rare in immunocompetent individuals; they are encountered most frequently in patients with haematological or lymphatic malignancies or AIDS.

CANDIDA

Candidal oesophagitis is often seen in association

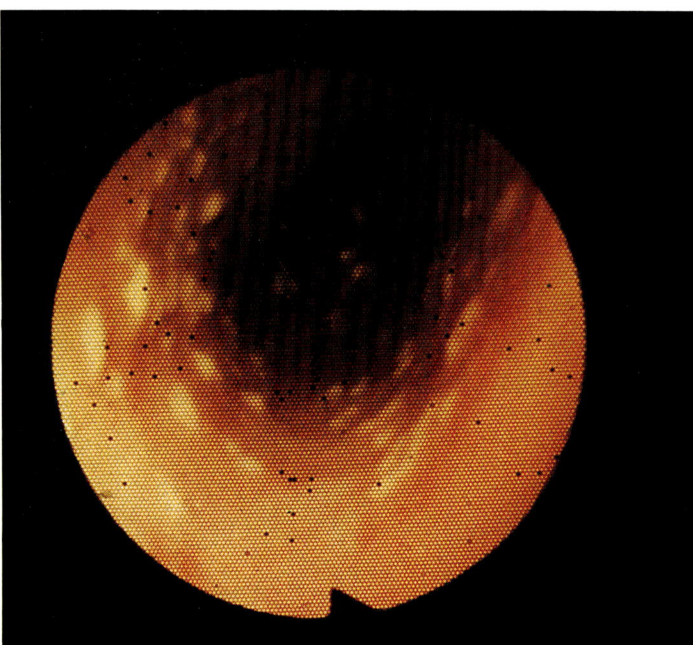

Fig. 1.1 Candida oesophagitis. Endoscopic view showing multiple cotton-wool plaques on the mucosa. This is a mild case, in which barium swallow might be normal. By courtesy of Dr J. Cunningham.

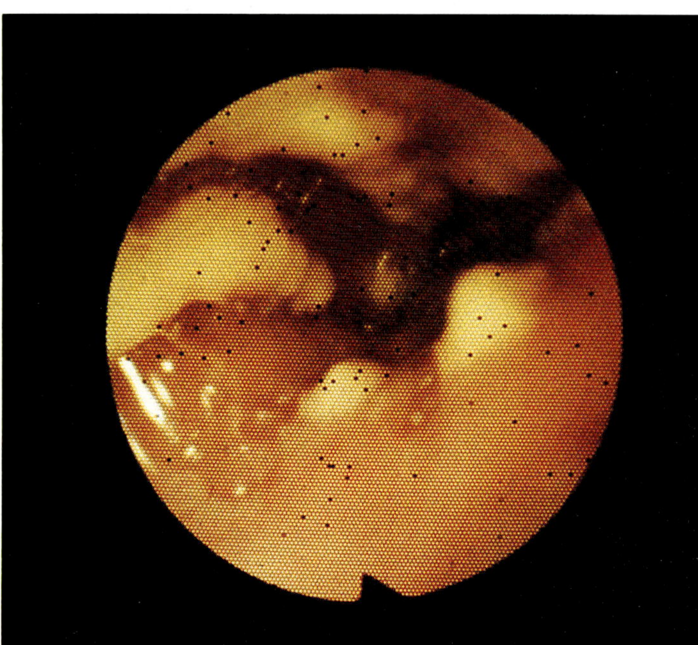

Fig. 1.2 Candida oesophagitis. A more advanced stage of severe oesophagitis with ulceration, showing discrete ulcers and thrush-like plaques on the mucosa. By courtesy of Dr J. Cunningham.

with extensive oral candidiasis (thrush), but approximately one-third of patients do not have thrush. The most common symptoms are pain on swallowing, a sensation of obstruction on swallowing and substernal chest pain. Endoscopic visualization of white plaques resembling thrush (Figs 1.1, 1.2 & 1.3), hyphal elements in cytological prepara-

tions made from scrapings (Fig. 1.4) and irregularity of the oesophageal mucosa resulting from ulceration (Figs 1.5 & 1.6) are also commonly found. Definitive diagnosis is best made by endoscopic biopsy, which reveals invasion of the mucosa by hyphal elements (Fig. 1.7). The stomach, small bowel and large bowel may also be involved, and in

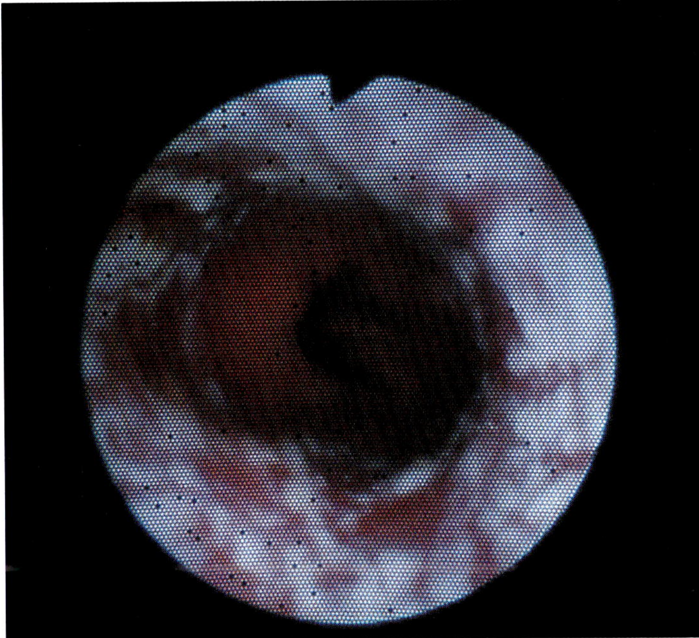

Fig. 1.3 Candida oesophagitis. Endoscopic view showing extensive areas of whitish exudate resembling the lesions of oral thrush. By courtesy of Dr I. Chesner.

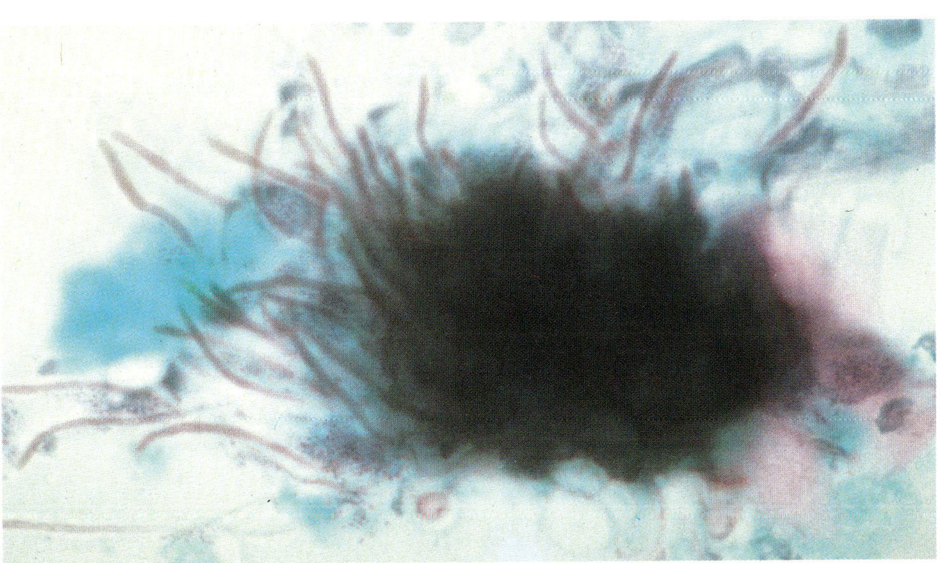

Fig. 1.4 A cytological preparation showing candidal hyphae growing outwards from a central fungal ball. ×900. Papanicolaou's stain. By courtesy of Dr E. Hudson.

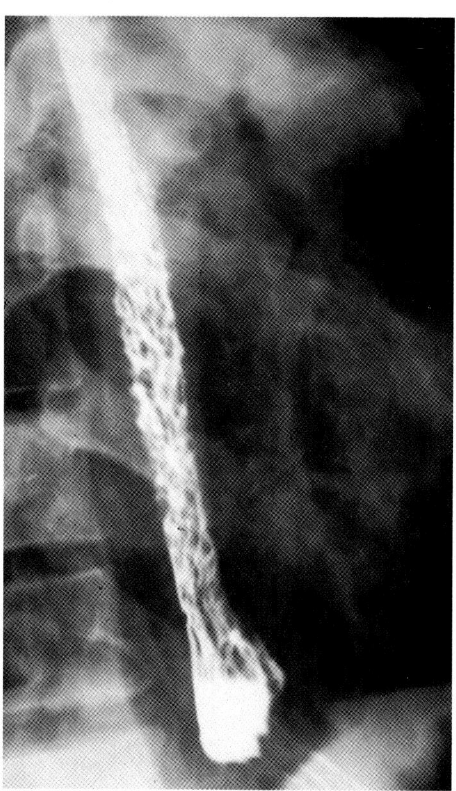

Fig. 1.5 Candida oesophagitis. Barium swallow showing multiple small ulcers, many of which contain barium, and narrowing of the oesophagus.

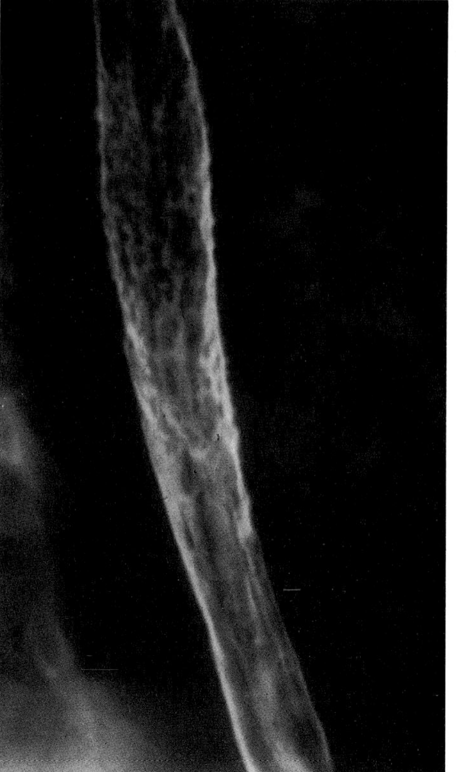

Fig. 1.6 Candida oesophagitis. Barium swallow showing multiple pinpoint ulcers. Note sawtooth pattern along lateral sides of oesophagus produced by barium remaining in the ulcers. Herpes simplex oesophagitis can exhibit a similar picture on barium swallow. By courtesy of Dr J. Cunningham.

severely immunocompromised patients concomitant infection with herpes simplex virus may be present. Oral nystatin often provides rapid relief of symptoms, but patients who fail to respond to this and those with severe infections should be treated with oral fluconazole or ketoconazole. Rarely therapy with amphotericin B given intravenously may be required. It may be impossible to completely eradicate oesophageal candidiasis in patients with AIDS; long-term suppression with fluconazole may be the best that can be achieved.

HERPES SIMPLEX VIRUS

Oesophagitis due to herpes simplex virus (HSV) is seen primarily in patients with AIDS, or those with haematological or lymphoreticular malignancies, or following organ transplantation. Pain and difficulty on swallowing are common features, and significant bleeding may occur. Endoscopy reveals ulceration and frequently vesicles similar to those seen in other infections of mucous membranes due to this virus (Figs 1.8 & 1.9). Unsuspected herpetic

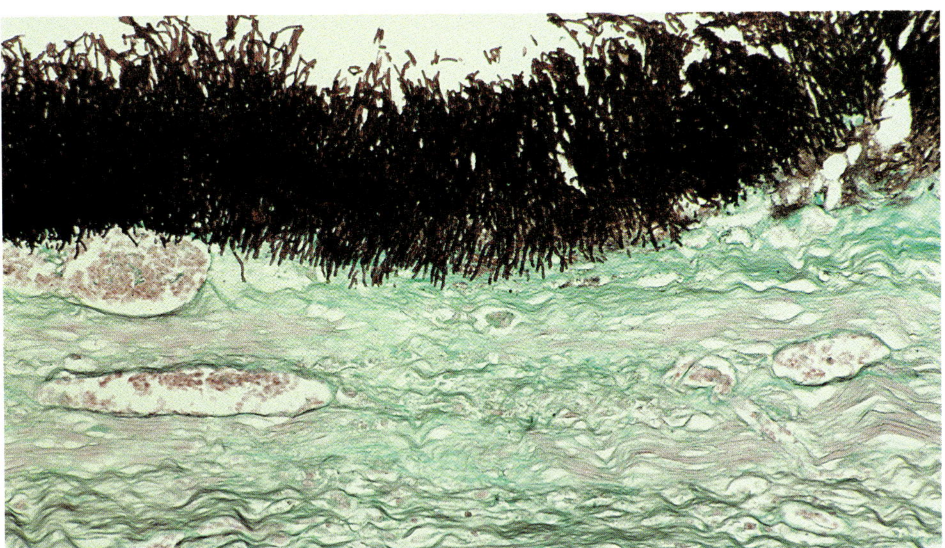

Fig. 1.7 Candida oesophagitis. Silver stain showing heavy infection of the mucosal surface by mycelial elements of *Candida*

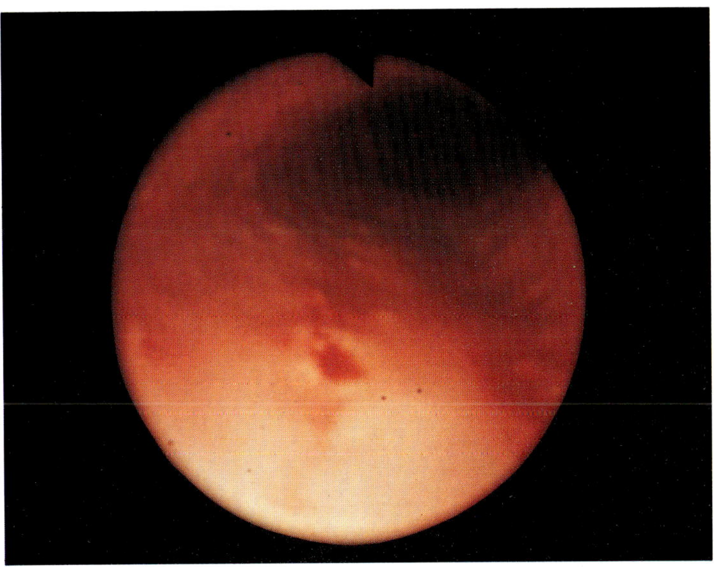

Fig. 1.8 Herpes simplex oesophagitis. Endoscopic view showing multiple pinpoint ulcers with haemorrhagic bases in a patient with severe odynophagia. By courtesy of Dr J. Cunningham.

oesophagitis is often found at autopsy, especially in patients who have had nasogastric tubes in place shortly before death. Prophylactic administration of acyclovir intravenously may prevent the development of progressive mucocutaneous and visceral herpes simplex infections in certain high risk individuals, such as HSV-seropositive recipients of bone marrow transplants. Acyclovir given intravenously is also highly effective in treatment of these infections.

OTHER INFECTIONS

Ulcerative oesophageal lesions, possibly due to direct infection with the HIV virus, have been observed in patients recently infected with this virus. In rare cases the oesophagus may be involved in disseminated infection with *Mycobacterium avium–intracellulare* in patients with AIDS (Fig. 1.10).

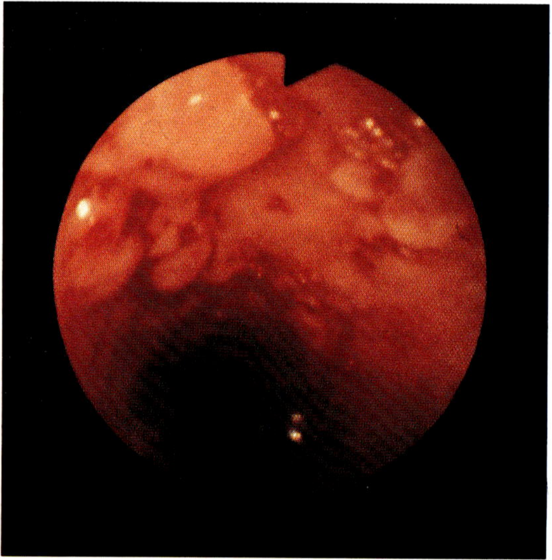

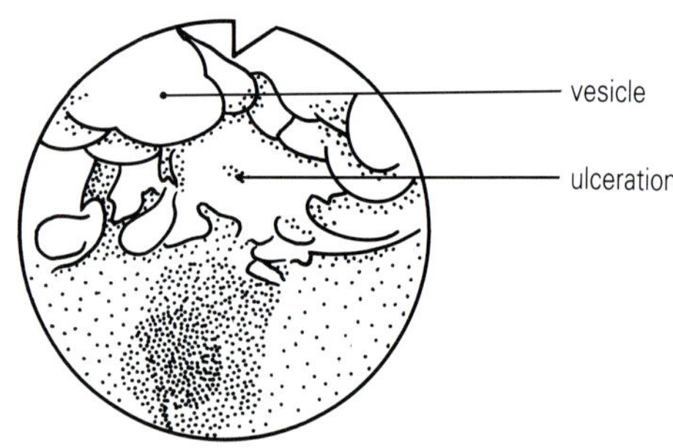

Fig. 1.9 Endoscopic view of oesophagitis due to herpes simplex virus showing herpetic vesicles and multiple ulcers.

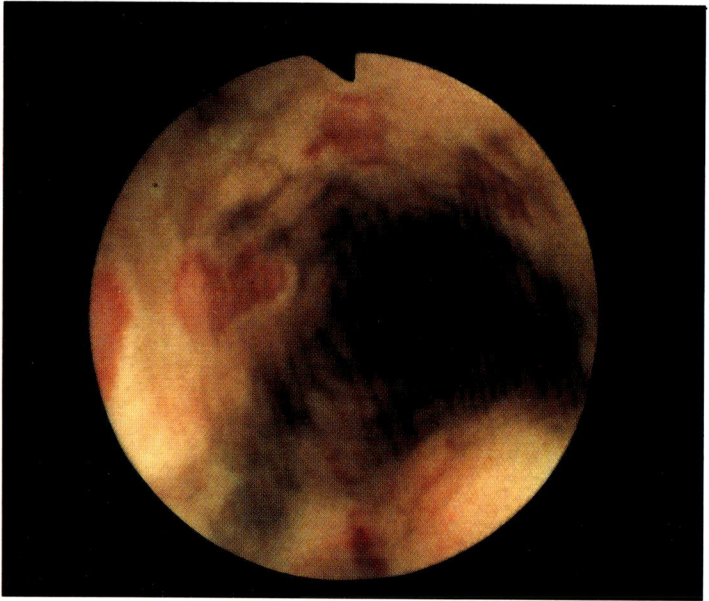

Fig. 1.10 Oesophagitis due to *Mycobacterium avium–intracellulare*. Chronic ulcerations and patches of yellow exudate with a few islands of intact mucosa. By courtesy of Dr J. Cunningham.

INFECTIOUS GASTRITIS

Two important causes of gastritis are *Helicobacter pylori* (formerly *Campylobacter pylori*) and cytomegalovirus.

HELICOBACTER PYLORI

During the last few years a large body of evidence has accumulated which implicates *H. pylori* as an aetiological agent in idiopathic or type B gastritis (Fig. 1.11), non-ulcer dyspepsia and duodenal ulcer. This organism is a microaerophilic, curved or spiral, gram-negative rod which produces a potent urease, an enzyme which catalyses the hydrolysis of urea to carbon dioxide and ammonia. The bacteria live in the mucous layer overlying the gastric epithelium and apparently do not invade the tissues (Fig. 1.12). The ability of these acid-susceptible organisms to survive in the stomach may depend upon the protective effect of the mucous layer and upon local neutralization of gastric acid by ammonia (produced by the action of urease). At the present time, diagnosis of *H. pylori* infection is made by isolation of the organism from biopsy specimens, with visualization of the characteristic bacteria in histological sections stained with Gram's, silver, Giemsa or acridine orange stains, or

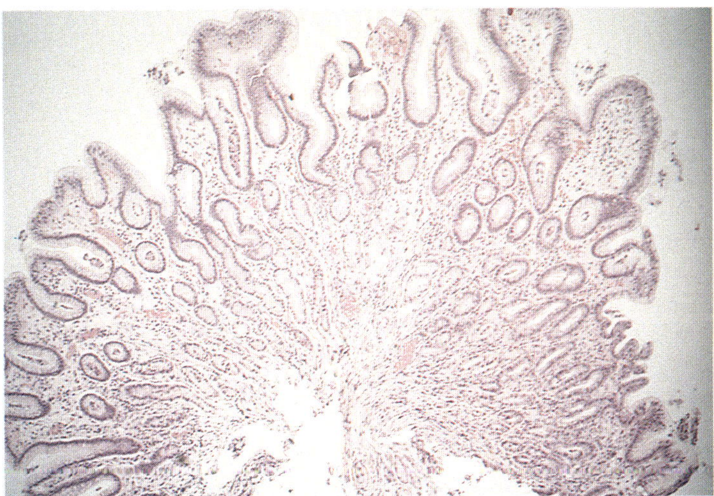

Fig. 1.11 *Helicobacter pylori* gastritis. Non-specific inflammatory changes in gastric mucosa associated with infection with *H. pylori*. By courtesy of Dr J. Newman.

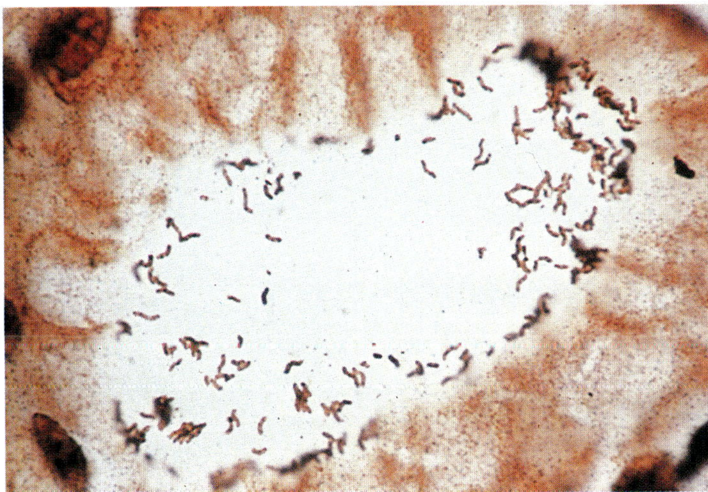

Fig. 1.12 *Helicobacter pylori* gastritis. Silver stain showing numerous comma-shaped organisms adhering to the mucosal surface. By courtesy of Dr A. M. Geddes.

demonstration of urease activity either in biopsy specimens (using the commercially available CLO test) or by means of the ^{14}C-urea breath test, which measures radiolabelled CO_2 released from urea by the action of urease, or by determination of serum antibodies to *H. pylori*. Sensitive immunofluorescent methods, using monoclonal antibodies for demonstration of the organisms in gastric biopsy material, are being developed.

H. pylori organisms are susceptible to a number of different antimicrobial agents including amoxicillin, nitrofurans, metronidazole and bismuth salts. An effective regimen has been a combination of bismuth with either tetracycline or ampicillin, administered orally for 4 weeks, with metronidazole for the first 2 weeks. When the organism is successfully eradicated by treatment, symptoms remit and the histopathological abnormalities improve. Reappearance of the organisms is followed by clinical and histopathological relapse.

CYTOMEGALOVIRUS

Infection of the gastrointestinal tract by cytomegalovirus (CMV) occurs commonly in patients who are severely immunocompromised. Gastritis is the most common type of gastrointestinal infection with the virus but any level of the gastrointestinal tract may be involved. The most common symptoms are epigastric pain, anorexia, fever, nausea and vomiting, diarrhoea and gastrointestinal bleeding. Diagnosis is made by upper endoscopy, which reveals nodular and/or erosive gastritis, and biopsy. The tissue specimens should be examined for inclusion bodies, CMV antigen-specific immunofluorescence and culture for CMV. Ganciclovir administered intravenously (5 mg/kg twice daily for a minimum of 2 weeks) is effective in the treatment of CMV infection of the gastrointestinal tract.

Chapter 2

Bacterial Enteric Infections

Bacteria may produce diarrhoea by production of toxins, by invasion of the intestinal mucosa, or by certain other mechanisms which involve close adherence of the bacteria to the intestinal mucosal cell (*Escherichia coli* – see below).

Toxins may include classic enterotoxins, which cause fluid secretion into the gut by stimulating adenylate cyclase or guanylate cyclase activity, as well as more general cytotoxins. Enterotoxins may be detected by their ability to produce fluid secretion in the isolated intestinal loop of the rabbit (Fig. 2.1) and by the Chinese hamster ovary cell and Y-1 adrenal cell assays (Fig. 2.2). Classic enterotoxins such as cholera toxin produce an essentially pure biochemical lesion, with virtually no histopathological effects on the intestinal mucosa.

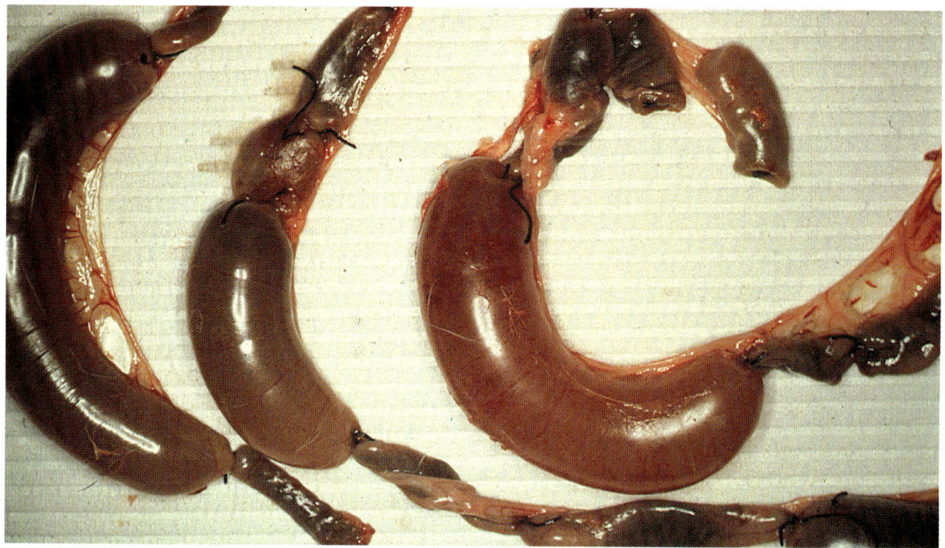

Fig. 2.1 *Escherichia coli* diarrhoea. Rabbit loop assay showing massive secretion of fluid into ligated intestinal loops which have been injected with *E. coli* enterotoxin. By courtesy of Dr H. L. DuPont.

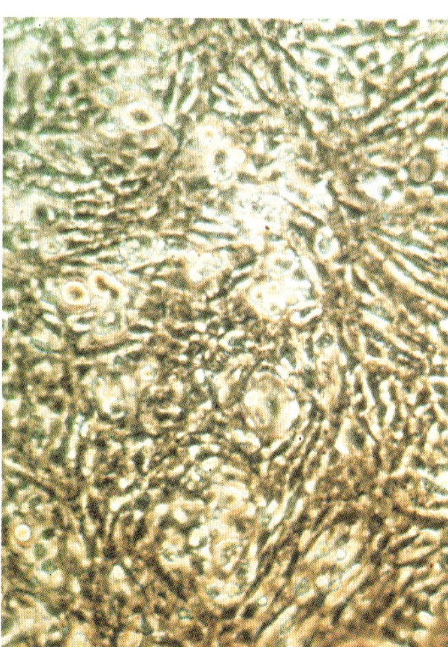
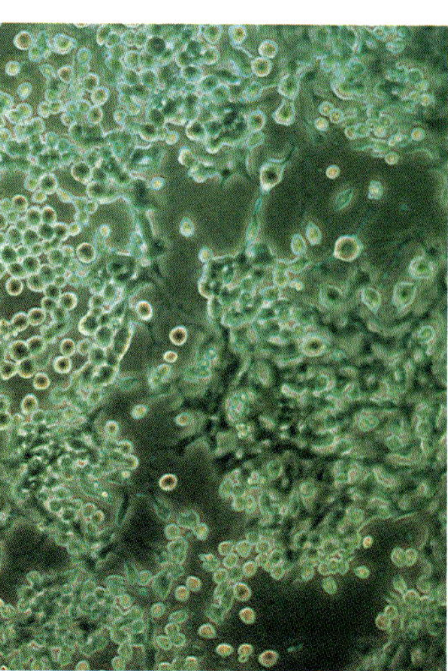

Fig. 2.2 Bacterial diarrhoea. Y-1 adrenal cell assay for *E. coli* LT enterotoxin, showing normal cells (left) and cells after exposure to LT toxin (right). Note disruption of monolayer and rounding up of cells. By courtesy of Dr H. L. DuPont.

Some important enterotoxin-producing organisms are *Vibrio cholerae, E. coli,* and *Clostridium perfringens* type A. Cytotoxins are produced by *Shigella dysenteriae* type 1, *Clostridium difficile* and certain *E. coli* serotypes (e.g. 0:157), among others.

Invasive organisms penetrate through the epithelium of the bowel into the lamina propria, and sometimes beyond, where they stimulate an intense acute inflammatory reaction with accumulation of large numbers of polymorphonuclear leucocytes (Fig. 2.3). This direct damage to the intestinal mucosa and the accompanying inflammatory reaction results in the presence of blood, mucus and inflammatory cells (polymorphonuclear leucocytes) in the stool (dysentery) (Fig. 2.4). The invasiveness of these organisms is not limited to the

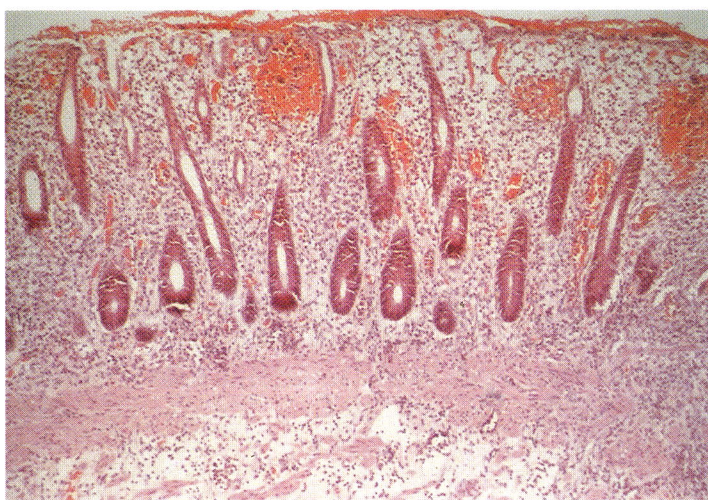

Fig. 2.3 Bacterial diarrhoea (*Campylobacter* spp.). Rectal biopsy showing marked mucosal oedema with polymorphonuclear leucocyte infiltration. Crypt degeneration has led to an attenuated appearance. H&E stain. By courtesy of Dr A. B. Price.

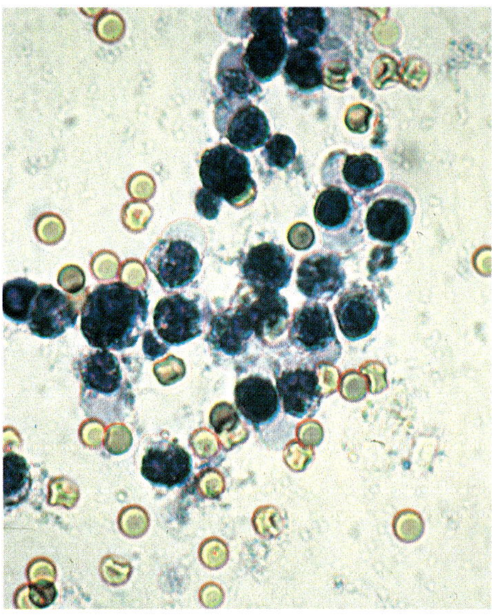

Fig. 2.4 Shigellosis. Polymorphonuclear and mononuclear leucocytes and red blood cells in the stool of a patient with shigellosis. Methylene blue wet mount under cover slip. By courtesy of Dr H. L. DuPont.

gut; invasiveness may be detected in cell cultures (Fig. 2.5) or by putting a drop of a culture of the organism into a rabbit's eye, where an intense keratoconjunctivitis is produced (Sereny test – Fig. 2.6). Virulence of both toxin-producing and invasive pathogens also depends upon the presence of adherence factors, which cause the bacteria to closely adhere to the mucosal cells (Fig. 2.7). Important invasive bacteria include *Shigella*, *Salmonella*, and *Campylobacter* species and certain strains of *E. coli.*

The clinical diseases produced by enterotoxigenic and invasive organisms differ in several respects; these are summarized in Fig. 2.8.

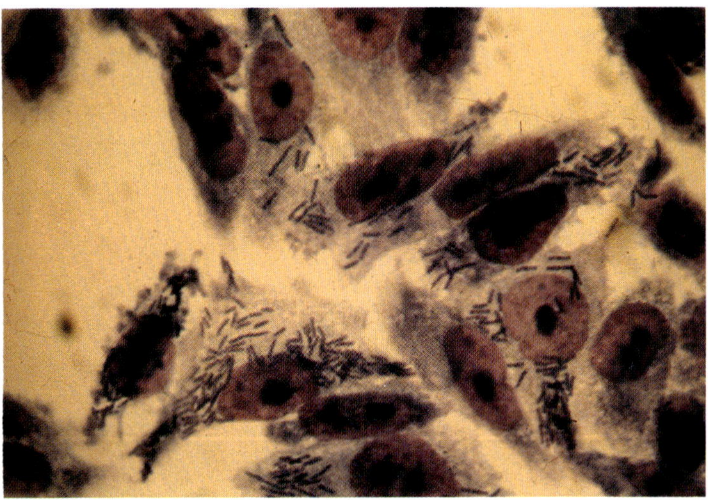

Fig. 2.5 Enteroinvasive *E. coli* infection. EIEC organisms invading HeLa cells *in vitro*. By courtesy of Dr S. Knutton.

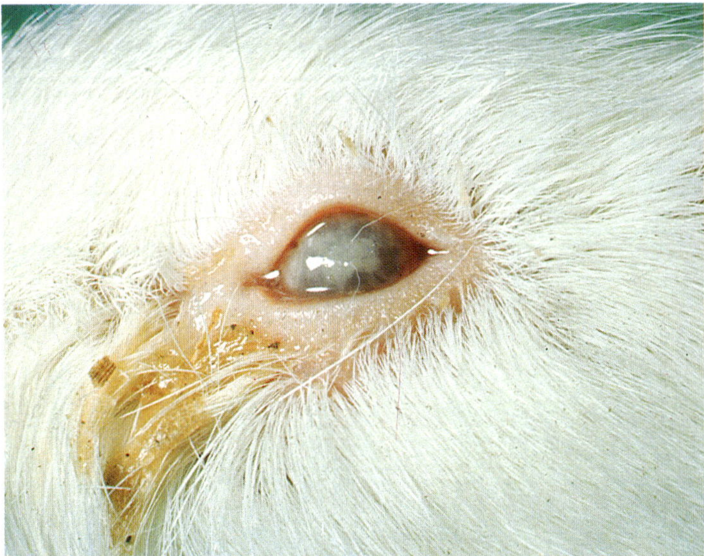

Fig. 2.6 Positive Sereny test. Keratoconjunctivitis in the rabbit produced by the instillation of shigella organisms. By courtesy of Dr H. L. DuPont.

VIBRIO INFECTIONS

Vibrio cholerae (cholera)

Cholera is the prototype of a diarrhoeal disease caused by an enterotoxin-producing microorganism. Although it has been known in India and other parts of Asia since ancient times, pandemic spread to Europe and other parts of the world first occurred early in the 19th century. Since that time the geographic distribution of cholera has expanded and contracted periodically for reasons which are poorly understood; at the time of writing (1991) the seventh recorded pandemic is in progress. The disease is most prevalent in southern Asia but small endemic foci exist in other areas of the world, including the coast of the Gulf of Mexico in the USA.

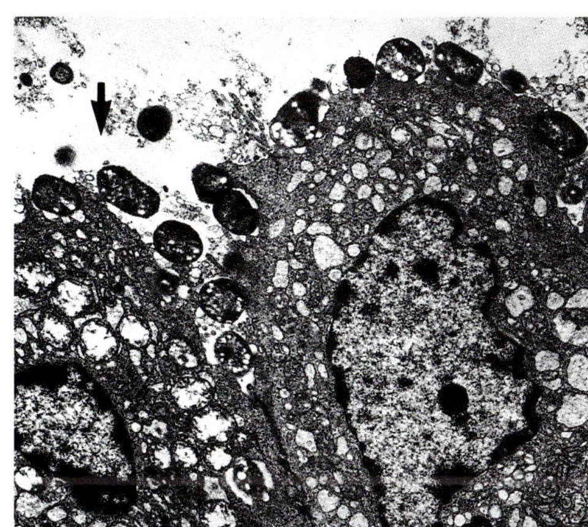

Fig.2.7 *Escheria coli* diarrhoea. Electron micrograph of enteropathogenic *E. coli* (arrowed) attached to mucosal epithelial cells of ileum. The microvillus border of the epithelial cells has been largely destroyed by bacteria and the cells show signs of degeneration. × 3000. By courtesy of Dr J. R. Cantey.

Clinical Disease Caused by Enterotoxigenic and Invasive Organisms	
Enterotoxigenic	**Invasive**
Severe watery diarrhoea, no dysentery	Dysentery (blood, mucus, PMN)
No fever	Fever
No systemic toxicity	Severe systemic toxicity
Minimal abdominal pain and cramping	Severe abdominal pain and cramping, tenesmus
Bacteria multiply in small bowel	Bacteria multiply in colon
No PMN leucocytes in stool	PMN leucocytes in stool
Response to non–absorbable antimicrobial agents	Response to absorbable and parenteral antibiotics

Fig. 2.8 Clinical disease caused by enterotoxigenic and invasive organisms.

Vibrio cholerae is a comma-shaped gram-negative rod, closely related to the other members of the Enterobacteriaceae. It exhibits rapid motility by means of a single polar flagellum. Classical cholera vibrios (01 serotype) agglutinate with Ogawa or Inaba antisera, but similar diarrhoeal disease may be due to non-01 (non-agglutinating) organisms. Man is the only known natural host for *V. cholerae*. As John Snow elegantly demonstrated in London in the 1840s and 1850s, during epidemics the disease spreads through contamination of the water supply. Direct faecal–oral transmission within households and contamination of food are also important.

Cholera toxin is a protein which has distinct binding and active subunits. The binding subunit binds to a specific receptor on the intestinal mucosal cell. The toxin stimulates the activity of cyclic AMP in the small intestinal mucosa, resulting in active secretion of chloride (Fig. 2.9) with secondary loss of sodium and water.

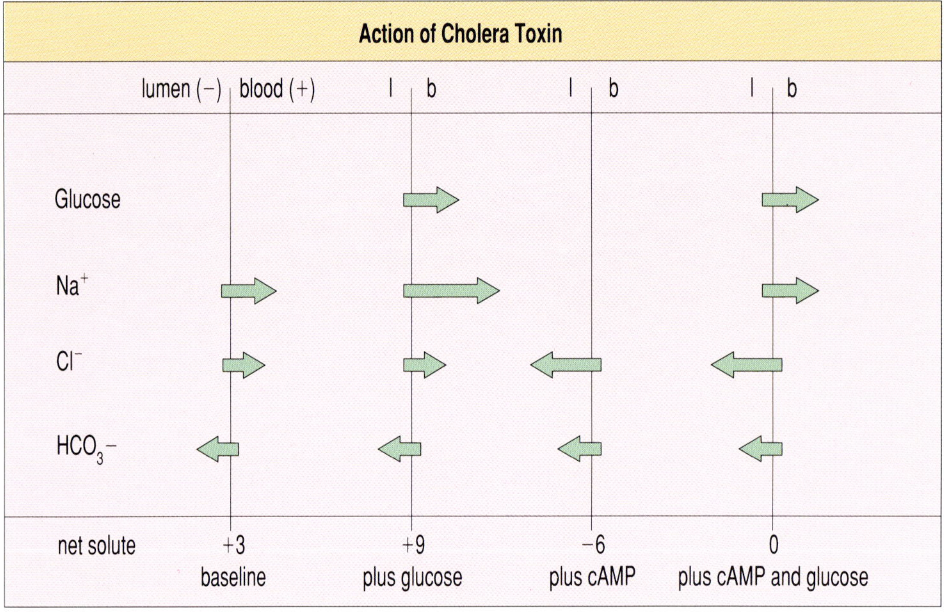

Fig. 2.9 Diagram showing action of cholera toxin on intestinal mucosa. The toxin stimulates the activity of cyclic AMP in the small intestinal mucosa, resulting in active secretion of chloride, with secondary loss of sodium and water. Glucose partially reverses the inhibition of sodium absorption. By courtesy of Dr M. Field.

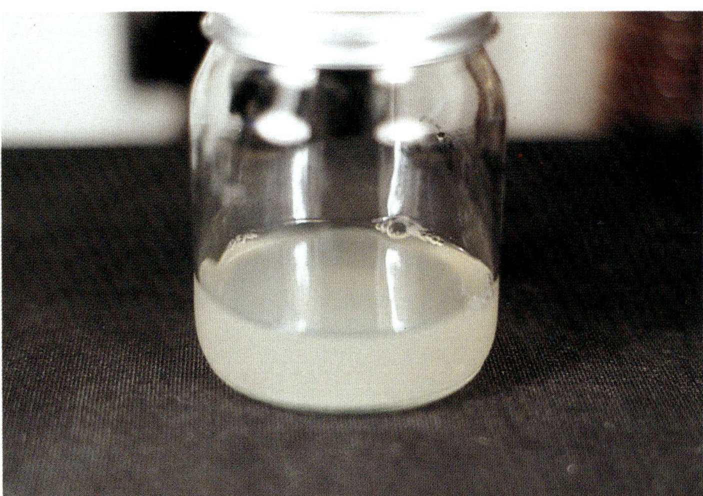

Fig. 2.10 Rice water stool in cholera. A typical large-volume watery stool excreted at the height of the illness. By courtesy of Dr A. M. Geddes.

The clinical picture of cholera consists of profound watery diarrhoea, with rapid depletion of water and electrolytes. At the height of the illness the voluminous watery stool is nearly colourless and contains flecks of mucus (the rice-water stool – Fig. 2.10). If water and electrolyte losses are replaced promptly the only other symptoms may be abdominal fullness and hyperperistalsis. If replacement is inadequate, hypovolaemia with shock, altered consciousness, renal failure, hypokalaemia and acidosis may develop. Patients with severe cholera may lose up to 20 litres of stool per day, a total of 100 litres during the 4–7 day course of the illness.

The most important aspect of treatment is rapid replacement of the lost water and electrolytes. In most patients this can be accomplished via the oral route, but in those who are severely ill or vomiting the intravenous route should be used. Glucose (or sucrose) must be added to oral replacement solutions since one phase of sodium absorption is glucose-dependent. Reasonably accurate estimates of the volume of fluid being lost can be made using the 'cholera cot' with a bucket and calibrated measuring stick (Fig. 2.11). Oral administration of an effective antibiotic such as tetracycline significantly shortens the duration of diarrhoea and reduces the total loss of fluid and electrolyte.

Bacteriological confirmation of the diagnosis of cholera may be made by culture of the stool or a rectal swab. Treatment must not be delayed until the bacteriological diagnosis is secured but should be initiated immediately, based upon the clinical picture.

Other vibrios

In recent years it has become apparent that non-01 cholera vibrios, sometimes known as non-agglutinable (NAG) vibrios, which are distributed worldwide in water sources, are capable of causing diarrhoeal disease. A few patients develop severe watery diarrhoea indistinguishable from classical cholera, but in most patients the diarrhoea is less severe and resembles the traveller's diarrhoea caused by enterotoxigenic strains of *E. coli*. These organisms are isolated on thiosulphate–citrate–bile salt–sucrose (TCBS) agar. Patients with mild diarrhoea need no treatment; in more severe illness replacement of lost fluid and electrolytes by oral or intravenous routes may be required. Whether or not antimicrobial agents shorten the course of illness in severe cases has not been established.

Of the true halophilic (salt-requiring) vibrios, the most important species is *Vibrio parahaemolyticus*. This organism is an extremely important cause of diarrhoeal disease in Japan and has recently been implicated in outbreaks of disease along the Atlantic and Gulf coasts of the USA and on Caribbean cruise ships. It occurs in coastal waters around the world and is probably a common cause of diarrhoea wherever inadequately cooked seafood is eaten. Nearly all cases are related to ingestion of seafood which has either been inadequately cooked or recontaminated with sea water containing the organism. *V. parahaemolyticus* produces an enterotoxin and also invades the bowel wall, stimulating an inflammatory reaction in the

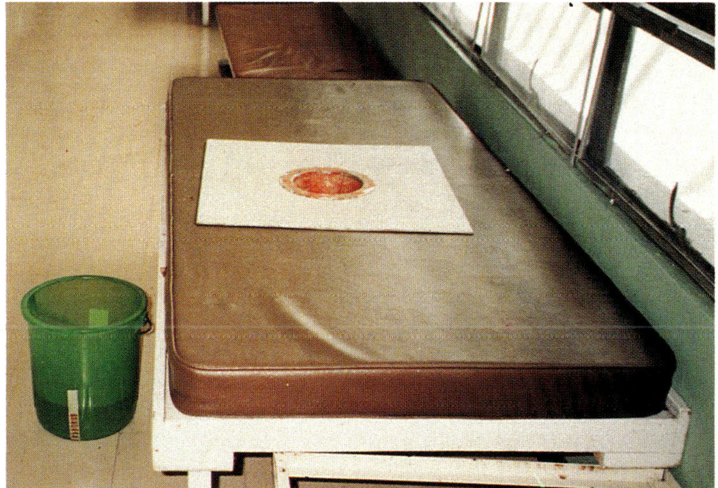

Fig. 2.11 A 'cholera cot' and bucket used for estimation of volume lost in stool. By courtesy of Dr S. Mehtar.

tissues. The incubation period is short, usually less than 24 hours, and the onset is abrupt with explosive watery diarrhoea and cramping abdominal pain. Fever, chills and headache may also be present. Halophilic vibrios grow poorly on standard culture media and isolation is best accomplished by inoculation onto TCBS agar.

Usually no treatment is required in *V. parahaemolyticus* infections, but occasionally replacement of fluid and electrolyte losses is indicated. The infection can be prevented by adequate cooking of seafood and avoidance of recontamination of cooked seafood by sea water containing the organism. Cooked seafood which is not eaten immediately should be refrigerated promptly.

Two other important halophilic vibrios, *V. vulnificus* and *V. alginolyticus,* are associated primarily with wound infections and sepsis rather than diarrhoeal disease.

ESCHERICHIA COLI INFECTIONS

Worldwide, diarrhoea-producing strains of *E. coli* are a major cause of diarrhoeal disease and, in young children, of mortality. As described below, several different pathogenetic mechanisms are involved (Fig. 2.12). There is only a rough correlation between pathogenetic type and serotype based on the O antigen (a lipopolysaccharide). Clinical features of the illnesses produced by the different types may also be dissimilar.

Enterotoxigenic *E. coli* (ETEC) adhere to microvilli of the small intestinal mucosa by means of pili or colonization factor antigens (Figs 2.13 & 2.14) and produce two distinct enterotoxins. The heat-labile toxin (LT) is a large protein of approximately 90 000 Da and is very similar to cholera toxin. Heat-stable toxins (ST) are small proteins of approximately 2000 Da which stimulate the guanylate cyclase of the mucosal cell, resulting in an increase in cyclic guanosine monophosphate (cGMP). ETEC strains are abundant in developing countries and are responsible for at least 50% of the cases of traveller's diarrhoea; they are rarely isolated from patients with diarrhoea in industrialized countries. Transmission is primarily via faecally contaminated food or water. The incubation period varies from 12 hours to 3 days. ETEC strains produce nausea, abdominal cramps and watery diarrhoea; fever and leucocytosis are usually absent.

Fig. 2.12 Pathogenetic types of *E. coli*.

Pathogenetic Types of *E. coli*
enterotoxigenic (ETEC)
enteroinvasive (EIEC)
non-enterotoxigenic, non-enteroinvasive
enteropathogenic (EPEC) (localized adherence)
enterohaemorrhagic (EHEC)
enteroaggregative (EAEC)
diffuse adherence

The illness is usually mild or only moderately severe, and lasts about 5 days on average.

Enteropathogenic *E. coli* (EPEC) adhere closely to intestinal cells (Fig. 2.15) but apparently do not produce adherence pili or LT or ST. There is loss of microvilli and aggregation of actin adjacent to sites of adherence (Fig. 2.16). The mechanism by which they produce diarrhoea is not completely

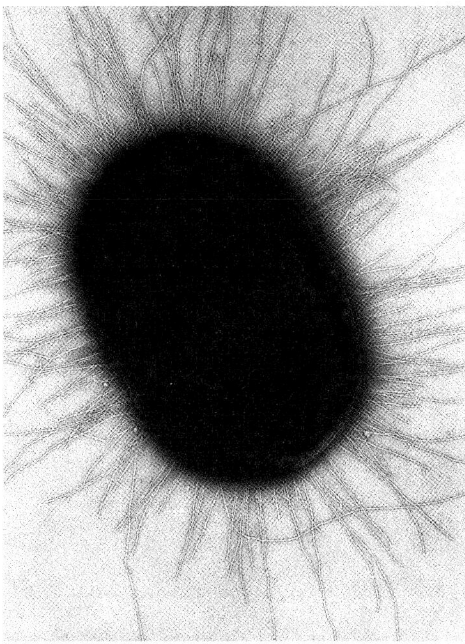

Fig. 2.13 Enterotoxigenic E. coli infection. Electron micrograph of the organism showing pili required for adherence to mucosal epithelial cells. By courtesy of Dr S. Knutton.

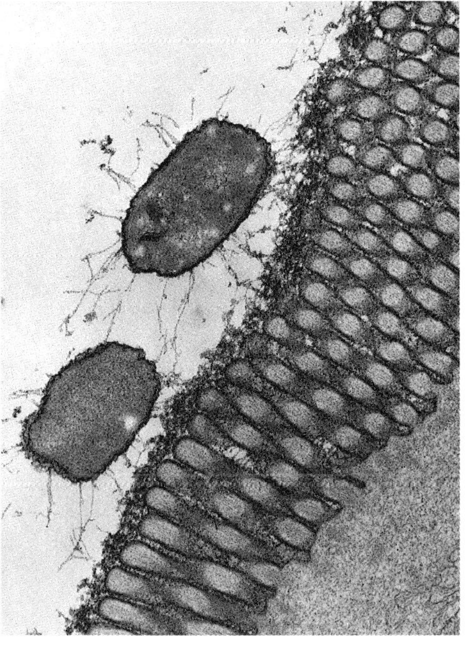

Fig. 2.14 Enterotoxigenic E. coli infection. Transmission electron micrograph showing bacteria adhering to the brush border of human intestinal mucosal cells. By courtesy of Dr S. Knutton.

understood. EPEC occur worldwide and have produced many epidemics, mainly involving young children. Diarrhoea often lasts for 10 days or longer, sometimes a month or more. In young children this may be associated with severe depletion of water and electrolytes.

Enterohaemorrhagic *E. coli* (EHEC) adhere closely to the mucosa of the distal ileum and proximal colon, but do not invade. They produce large amounts of Shiga-like toxins (Verotoxins), cytotoxic enterotoxins similar to the Shiga toxin originally found in strains of *Shigella dysenteriae* type 1, the Shiga bacillus (Fig. 2.17). Shiga-like toxin can often be detected in the diarrhoeal stool and may be responsible for the grossly bloody diarrhoea exhibited by these patients and, perhaps, for the associated haemolytic uraemic syndrome. EHECs were originally described in the USA in 1982 associated with ingestion of inadequately cooked hamburgers in fast-food restaurants. Most subsequent outbreaks have been associated with ingestion of contaminated food or milk, but person-to-person transmission

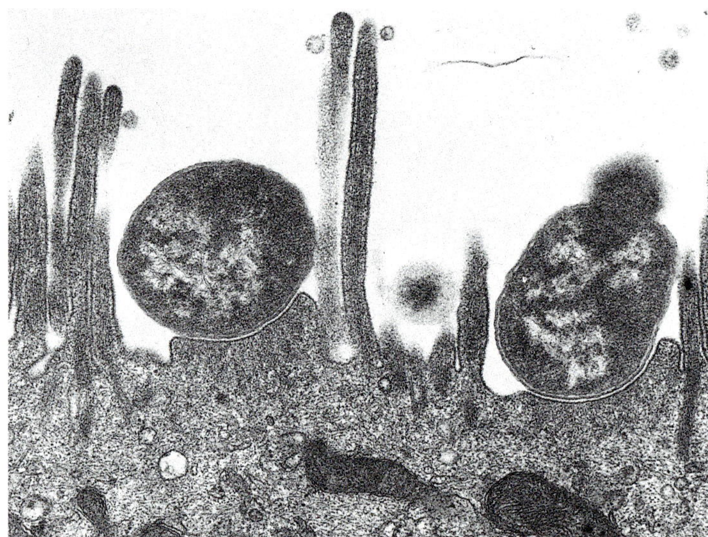

Fig. 2.15 Enteropathogenic *E. coli* infection. Electron micrograph showing close, localized adherence of bacteria to human intestinal mucosal cells and localized destruction of microvilli. By courtesy of Dr S. Knutton.

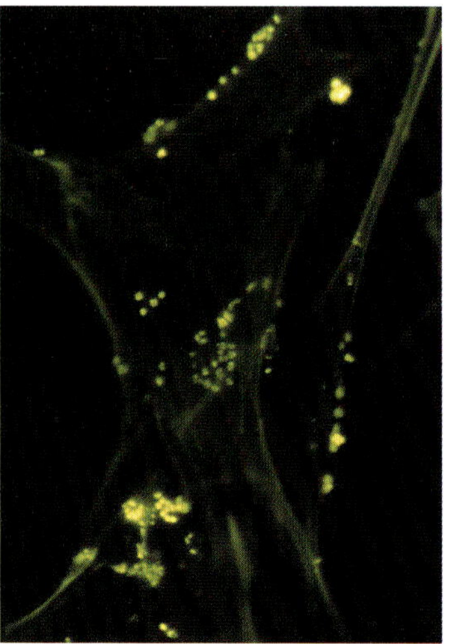
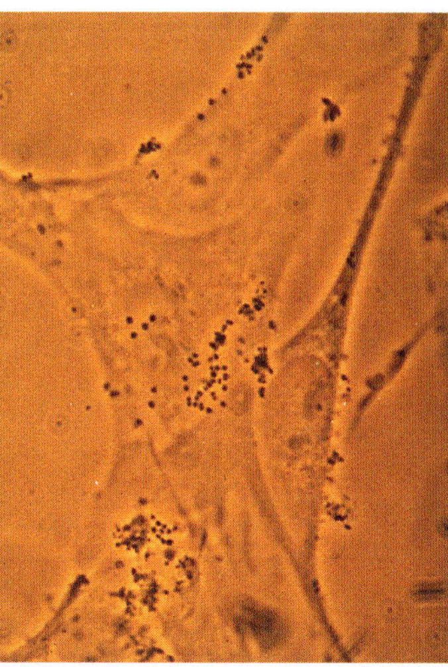

Fig. 2.16 Enteropathogenic *E. coli* infection. Fluorescent actin test specific for EPEC organisms. Left: Fluorescence microscopy showing aggregated actin. Right: Phase contrast microscopy showing location of bacteria. By courtesy of Dr S. Knutton.

can also occur. These organisms produce a distinctive clinical syndrome, ranging from non-bloody diarrhoea to full-blown haemorrhagic colitis, complicated in about 10% of cases by development of the haemolytic uraemic syndrome. The incubation period is longer than 8 days. Severe abdominal pain, marked abdominal distension and tenderness, especially in the right lower quadrant, are seen in most patients. X-rays show gas distending the small bowel, caecum and ascending colon and barium enema may show 'thumbprinting' of the caecum and ascending and transverse colon due to oedema and submucosal haemorrhage. On sigmoidoscopy and colonoscopy the mucosa may appear oedematous, friable and erythematous with haemorrhages and ulcerations, a picture which resembles ischaemic colitis. Patients with haemolytic uraemic syndrome exhibit deteriorating renal function, microangiopathic haemolytic anaemia and fibrin thrombi in glomerular capillaries (Fig. 2.18). Enteroinvasive *E. coli* (EIEC) produce diarrhoea by

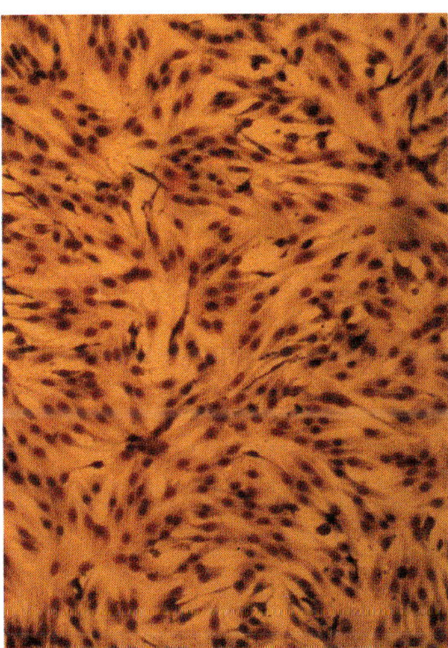

Fig. 2.17 Enterohaemorrhagic *E. coli* infection. Assay for Shiga-like toxin (Verotoxin) produced by EHEC (serotype 0:157). Left: Normal monolayer of Vero cells. Right: Destruction of Vero cells by the toxin. By courtesy of Dr S. Knutton.

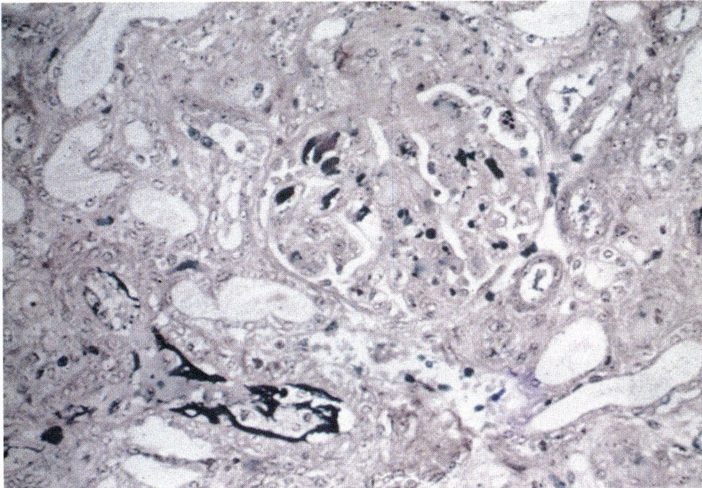

Fig. 2.18 Enterohaemorrhagic *E. coli* infection. Weigert stain showing fibrin 'thrombi' in glomerular capillaries in haemolytic uraemic syndrome. By courtesy of Dr H. R. Powell.

invading and destroying the mucosal epithelium of the distal ileum and colon (Fig. 2.19). This is a rare cause of diarrhoea, although it is occasionally responsible for large foodborne outbreaks, especially in tropical countries. The clinical picture of fever, systemic toxicity, cramping abdominal pain and dysentery is one that closely resembles shigellosis.

Specific microbiological diagnosis of diarrhoea due to *E. coli* is difficult and expensive. A small number of research or public health laboratories may be able to serotype *E. coli* isolates and identify EPEC strains; only a few research laboratories can carry out the specialized procedures required to identify the other types. DNA probes and assays to identify LT, ST, Shiga-like toxins and various adherence factors are being developed.

Most cases of diarrhoea due to *E. coli* are mild and adequate oral intake of fluids is the only treatment required. In more seriously ill patients intravenous administration of fluids and electrolytes may be necessary. Bismuth subsalicylate (Pepto-bismol) and antimotility agents (loperamide or diphenoxylate) are effective in reducing diarrhoea in patients without fever or dysentery. Presence of dysentery indicates invasive infection and these patients, as well as those with severe traveller's diarrhoea, should receive antibiotic therapy. Tetracycline, doxycycline, trimethoprim–sul-

phamethoxazole, furazolidone, and the quinolones (nalidixic acid and the fluoroquinolones) are all effective agents. A quinolone or furazolidone would be the best choice in areas where resistance to other antibiotics is prevalent.

SHIGELLOSIS (BACILLARY DYSENTERY)

Hippocrates provided the first description of dysentery; epidemics of bacillary dysentery are known to have occurred during military campaigns at least as long ago as the Peloponnesian Wars in the 5th century BC. Shigella organisms are highly adapted to man, the only natural host, and the minimum infectious dose is only about 200 organisms. Person-to-person transmission therefore occurs readily in crowded conditions, for example in military barracks, prisons, asylums, institutions for the mentally retarded and day-care centres. Shigella infections occur most frequently in infants and young children, but secondary spread within the household to other children and adults is common. The disease is most prevalent in tropical countries, and unsatisfactory conditions of hygiene and poor nutrition increase the incidence and severity. The peak incidence is during summer. Although most spread is person-to-person via contamination of the hands with infected faeces, outbreaks due to contamination of food or water supplies have occurred

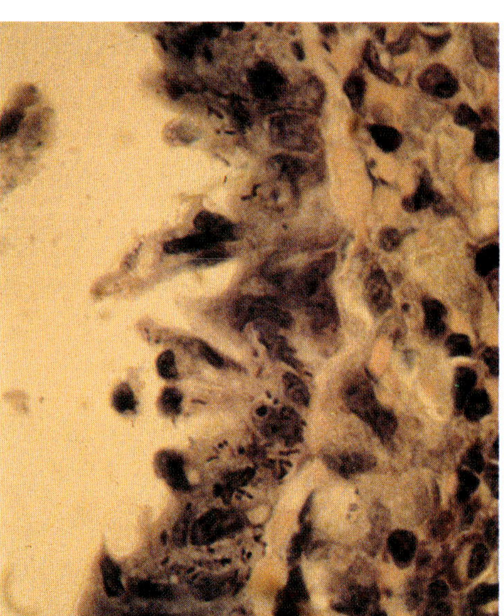
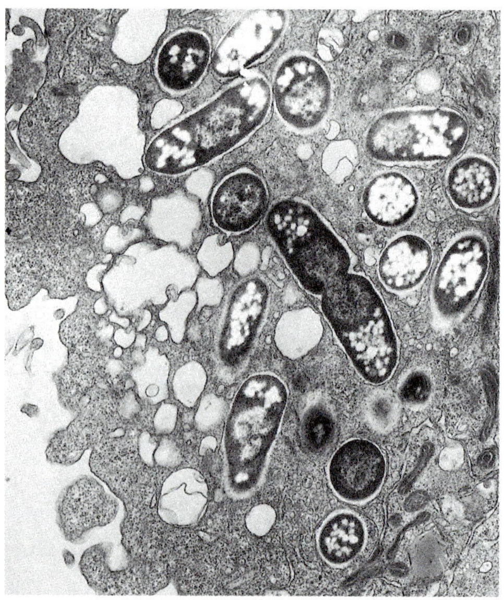

Fig. 2.19 Enteroinvasive *E. coli* infection. Invasion of mucosal layer of the intestine by *E. coli* organisms. There is necrosis of the mucosal layer at the site of invasion (left). Transmission electron micrograph showing enteroinvasive *E. coli* organisms within HEp-2 cell (right). By courtesy of Dr S. Knutton.

(e.g. on cruise ships) and there is good evidence that the organisms can be transmitted by flies.

The geographic distribution of each of the four species of shigella (*S. dysenteriae, S. flexneri, S. sonnei* and *S. boydii*) differs significantly. In general, *S. dysenteriae* is common only in impoverished tropical countries. In many less developed countries infection with *S. flexneri* predominates. In the most highly industrialized countries of northern Europe and North America, the majority of infections are caused by *S. sonnei. S. boydii* is the least common of the four species, but is endemic in a few countries in southern Europe.

Following ingestion, shigella organisms multiply in the distal small bowel and elicit symptoms of watery diarrhoea, cramping abdominal pain, fever, headache and other signs of systemic toxicity. In infants and young children hyperpyrexia and seizures may occur. Seizures and other neurological abnormalities may be due to Shiga or Shiga-like toxins. When the organism reaches the colon and invades the epithelium it multiplies primarily in the lamina propria, destroying the overlying mucosa (Fig. 2.20). Shigellas rarely penetrate beyond the mucosa, and bacteraemia is extremely rare. Sigmoidoscopy may reveal hyperaemia and a whitish exudate, and in severe cases an extensive

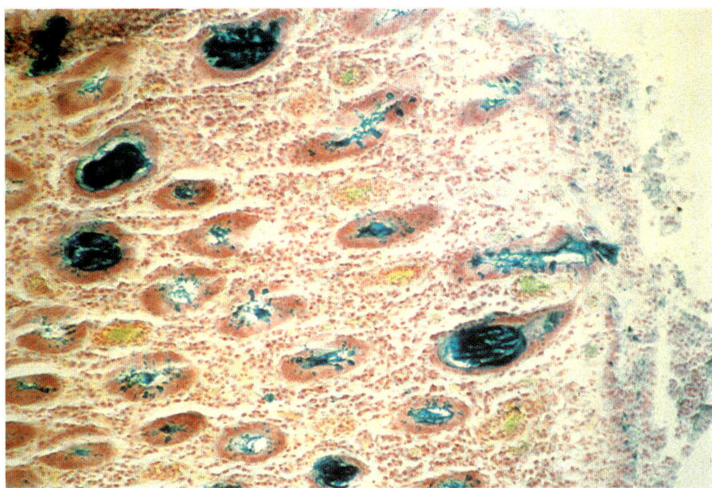

Fig. 2.20 Severe shigellosis. Histology of colon showing disrupted epithelium covered by pseudomembrane and interstitial infiltration. Mucin glands have uniformly discharged and goblet cells are empty. Colloidal iron stain. By courtesy of Dr R. H. Gilman.

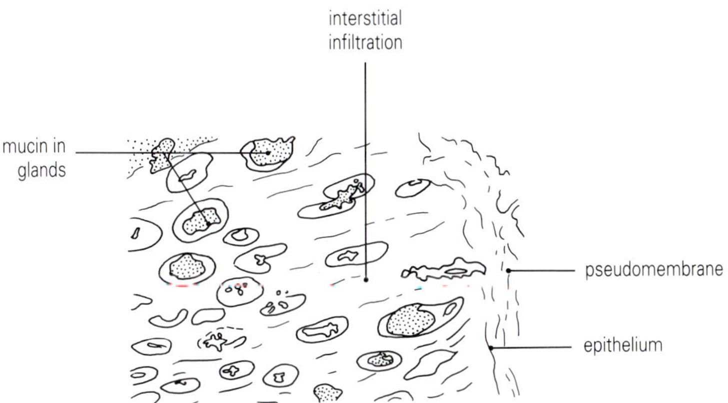

pseudomembranous colitis may be present (Figs 2.21 & 2.22). On histopathological examination microabscesses are seen which sometimes coalesce and cause sloughing, resulting in mucosal ulceration. At this stage the signs and symptoms reflect the invasion of the colonic wall; the patient experiences cramping abdominal pain, especially in the left lower quadrant, tenesmus and dysentery (blood, mucus and pus in the stool). If a fleck of mucus is mixed with a drop of saline and methylene blue stain and examined under a cover slip, large numbers of polymorphonuclear leucocytes are usually found (see Fig. 2.4). Many patients with shigellosis exhibit large numbers of band forms in the differential leucocyte count, up to 50% of the total number of leucocytes. Most patients recover within a few days to a week. Organisms may be excreted in the faeces from 1–4 weeks after recovery; long-term intestinal carriage rarely occurs.

Microbiological diagnosis of shigellosis depends upon isolation of the lactose-positive, gram-negative rods from a stool specimen or rectal swab. Organisms are most abundant and therefore easiest to isolate early in the course of the illness. The specimen should be inoculated into culture media as soon as it is obtained. The ideal method is to plate a rectal swab directly (at the bedside) onto mildly inhibitory media and also onto more inhibitory media.

Antibiotic treatment shortens the clinical course of the illness and reduces the duration of faecal excretion of shigellas. Antibiotics that are well absorbed following oral administration are best, since the organisms are located within the tissues of

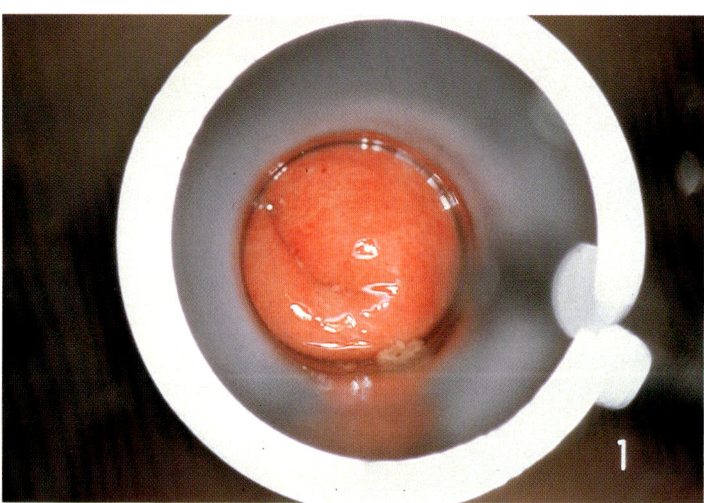

Fig. 2.21 Shigellosis. Sigmoidoscopic view of colonic mucosa in a mild case of infection due to *Shigella flexneri*. Note the thin whitish exudate, which is made up of fibrin and polymorphonuclear leucocytes. By courtesy of Dr R. H. Gilman.

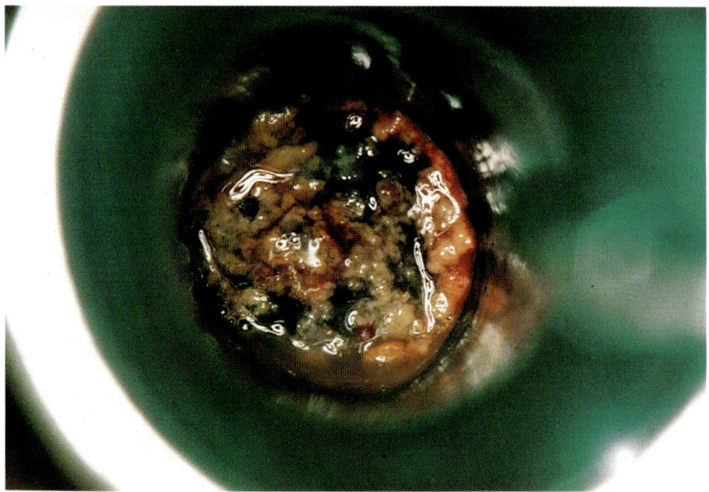

Fig. 2.22 Shigellosis. Sigmoidoscopic view of colonic mucosa in a fatal case of infection with *Shigella dysenteriae* type 1 showing extensive pseudomembranous colitis. By courtesy of Dr R. H. Gilman and Dr F. Koster.

the intestinal mucosa. Ampicillin, tetracyclines, trimethoprim–sulphamethoxazole, furazolidone, nalidixic acid and the fluoroquinolones are all effective against susceptible shigella strains, but resistance to the first three agents is now widespread in many tropical countries. Administration of anti-motility agents is contraindicated in shigellosis, as they may interfere with elimination of the organisms by peristalsis.

SALMONELLOSIS

Salmonella organisms are serologically extremely diverse, but may be grouped into three 'species':
1. *S. typhi* – causes typhoid fever, an 'enteric fever'
2. *S. choleraesuis* – often causes a septic, bacteraemic illness with focal metastatic infection
3. *S. enteritidis* (more than 1800 serotypes) – usually causes a self-limited enterocolitis, but certain serotypes may also cause enteric fever and other syndromes.

SALMONELLA TYPHI

S. typhi is exclusively a human pathogen, and is highly adapted to man. It causes typhoid fever, an enteric fever syndrome in which diarrhoea is rarely a prominent manifestation. Most infections with *S. typhi* are acquired by ingestion of contaminated water, food or milk. Since man is the only source of *S. typhi*, it is possible to control typhoid fever by eliminating human faecal contamination from water supplies and foods. In industrialized countries most cases of typhoid fever occur either in immigrants from endemic areas or in people returning from holidays in areas where the disease is common. It is also occasionally seen in young children who have acquired the disease from an older member of the household who is a chronic carrier of *S. typhi* and prepares food for the family. This has led to the aphorism 'to culture the grandmother'.

The organism invades the intestinal epithelium, with prominent involvement of Peyer's patches (Fig. 2.23) and production of ulceration (Figs 2.24

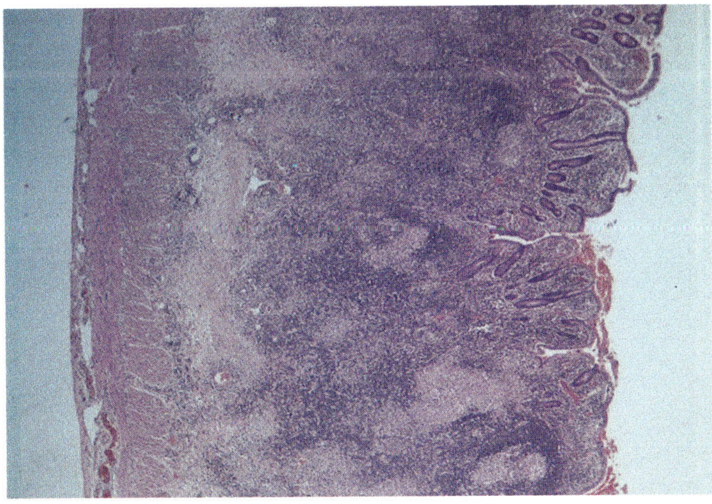

Fig. 2.23 Histological appearance of the ileum in typhoid fever showing prominent lymphoid hyperplasia and small slit-like ulcers. At this magnification the initial impression is one of lymphoma. ×10. H&E stain.

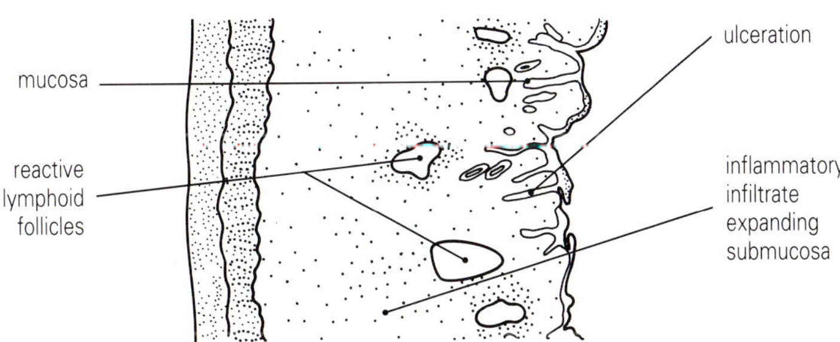

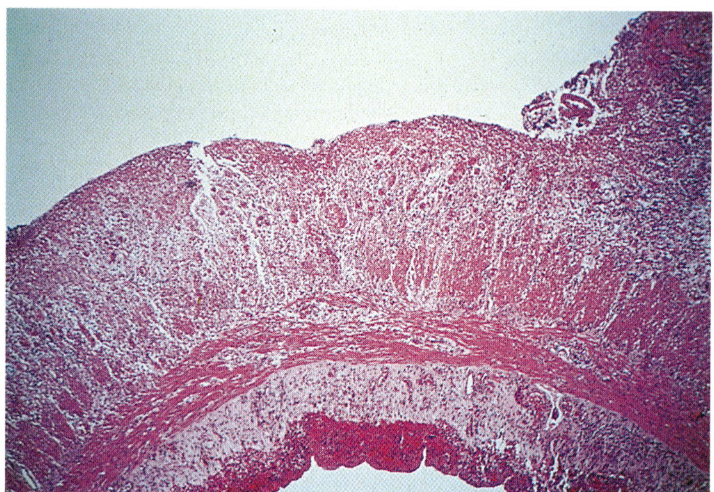

Fig. 2.24 Typhoid fever. Section of ileum showing a typhoid ulcer. There is a transmural inflammatory reaction, focal areas of necrosis and a fibrinous exudate on the serosal surface. H&E stain. By courtesy of Prof. M. S. R. Hutt.

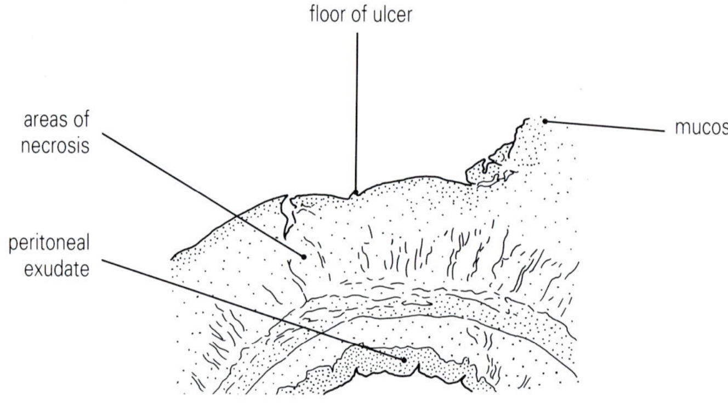

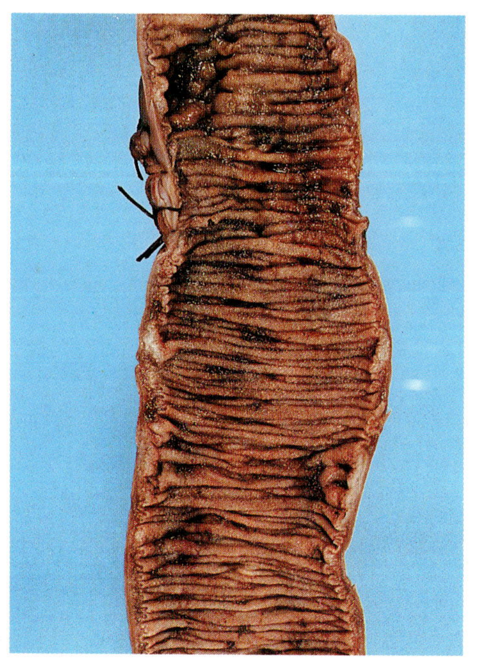

Fig. 2.25 Typhoid fever. Numerous ulcers of the small intestine overlying hyperplastic lymphoid follicles (Peyer's patches). By courtesy of Dr J. Newman.

& 2.25). The inflammatory infiltrate in the mucosa is composed primarily of mononuclear cells (Fig. 2.26) and large numbers of mononuclear cells may be present in the faeces (Fig. 2.27). Following an incubation period of 10–14 days, fever, malaise, anorexia, headache and myalgias develop. Remittent fever increases to a level of approximately 40°C by the end of the first week of illness

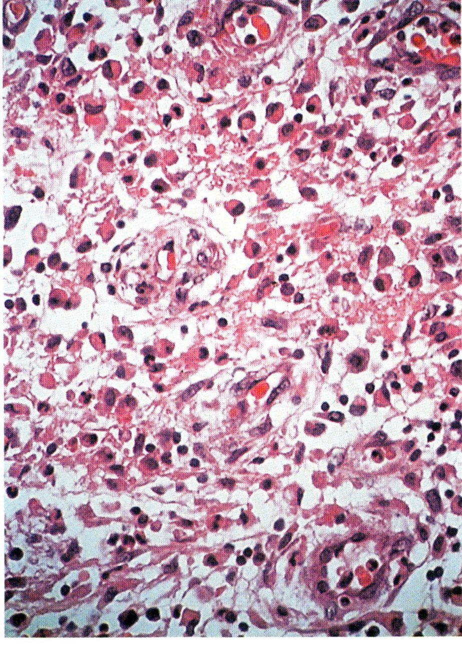

Fig. 2.26 Typhoid fever. Fig. 2.24 at higher magnification showing the typical mononuclear inflammatory cell response in the base of a typhoid ulcer. Most of the cells are macrophages. Note the absence of neutrophils. H&E stain. By courtesy of Prof. M. S. R. Hutt.

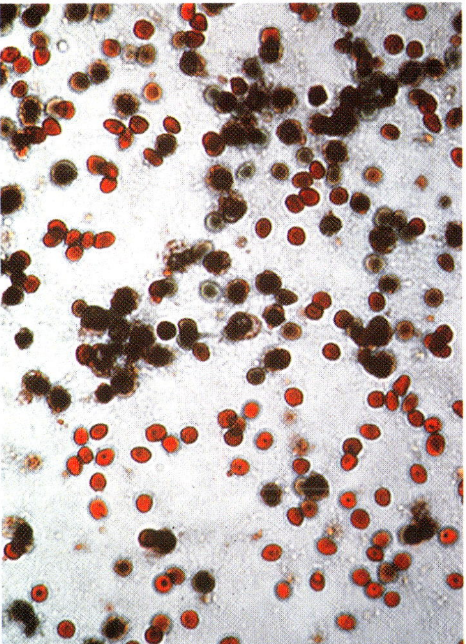

Fig. 2.27 Typhoid fever. Mononuclear cells and red blood cells in the stool. Trichrome stain. By courtesy of Dr H. L. DuPont.

(Fig. 2.28). Cough, sore throat, abdominal pain, chills, nausea and vomiting, diarrhoea or constipation, epistaxis, confusion, lethargy and delirium may also occur. The patient usually appears acutely ill. Rose spots, erythematous maculopapular lesions 2–4 mm in diameter that blanch on pressure, often appear on the abdomen (Figs 2.29 & 2.30). Usually less than 12 lesions are present, and they disappear within a few days. Enlargement of the liver and/or spleen is observed in approximately 50% of patients. Untreated, typhoid fever usually resolves 3–4 weeks after onset of illness. Effective antibiotic

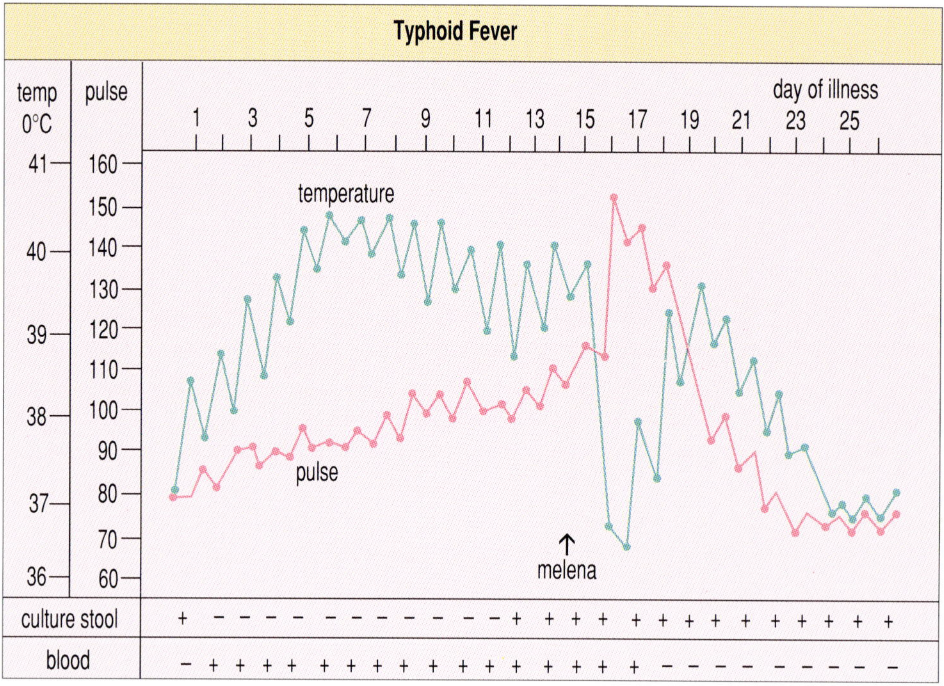

Fig. 2.28 Typhoid fever. Chart showing temperature, pulse rate and bacteriological findings in a patient whose course was complicated by a massive haemorrhage. Note the initial bradycardia with stepwise increase in the pulse rate. By courtesy of Dr H. L. DuPont.

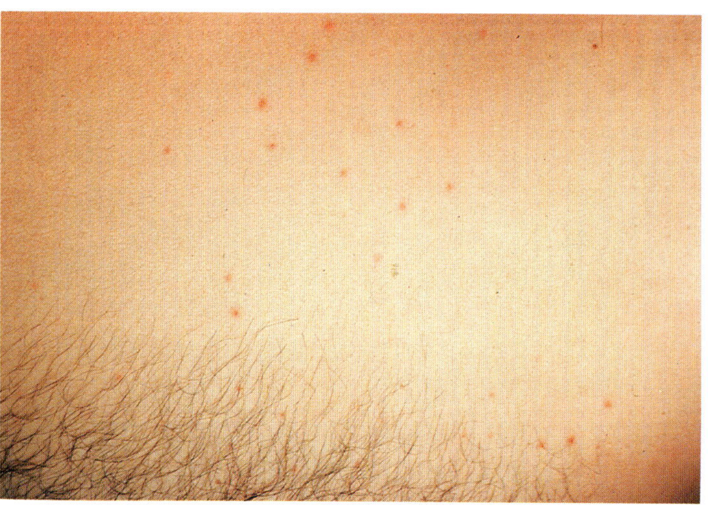

Fig. 2.29 Typhoid fever. Rose spots, small maculopapular erythematous lesions usually seen on the abdomen. By courtesy of Dr A. M. Geddes.

therapy shortens the duration of illness and fever usually resolves 3–5 days after the institution of therapy. Serious complications, including perforation, haemorrhage and toxic megacolon (Fig. 2.31) are rare in patients receiving appropriate therapy. Clinical relapse occurs in approximately 10% of patients, treated or untreated; the relapse rate may be significantly increased in patients treated with chloramphenicol.

Excretion of the organism in the faeces for several weeks after recovery is common, but a chronic carrier state (excretion of the organism for more than one year) develops in up to 3% of patients with typhoid fever. Older age, female sex and presence of disease of the biliary tract, especially cholelithiasis (hence the 'fat female over 40') are all factors associated with increased incidence of chronic biliary carriage of *S. typhi*. Stones in the urinary tract

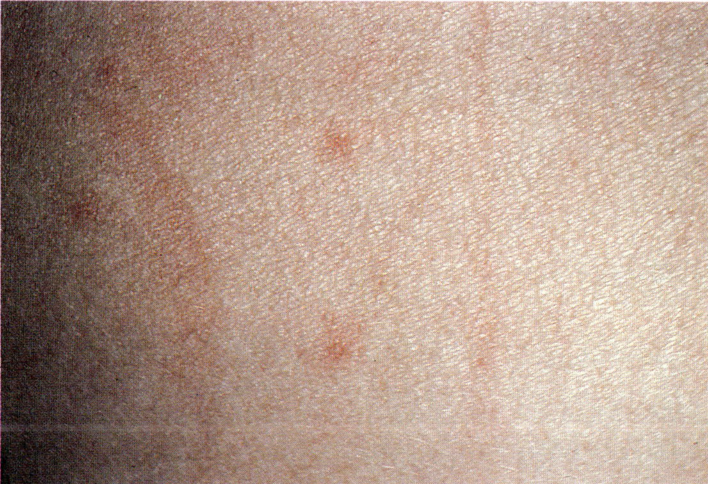

Fig. 2.30 Typhoid fever. Close-up view of rose spots.

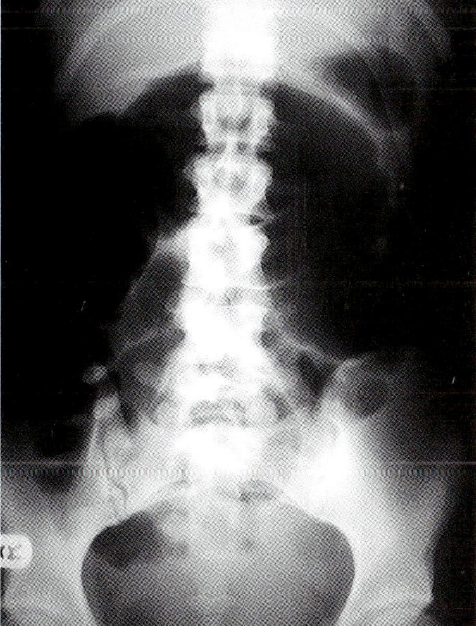

Fig. 2.31 Salmonellosis. Plain abdominal x-ray film showing distended, gas-filled colon in a patient with toxic megacolon.

and infection of the bladder with *Schistosoma haematobium* are associated with chronic urinary carriage of *S. typhi.*

Chloramphenicol, ampicillin, amoxicillin, trimethoprim-sulphamethoxazole and ciprofloxacin, given in full dosage for at least 2 weeks, have all been effective in the treatment of typhoid fever. Many other antimicrobial agents, effective *in vitro* against *S. typhi*, have not proved to be effective clinically. For treatment of the chronic carrier state in a patient who has a normally functioning gall bladder without evidence of cholelithiasis, ampicillin (4–6 per day) combined with probenecid (2 g per day), given as four oral doses per day for six weeks, is the treatment of choice. If gallbladder disease is present, and if there is no contraindication to surgery, cholecystectomy should be performed. Even without cholecystectomy about 25% of chronic *S. typhi* carriers with biliary tract disease can be cured with ampicillin. Trimethoprim–sulphamethoxazole plus rifampin and ciprofloxacin given as a single agent have also been effective in the treatment of chronic carriers of *S. typhi.*

Other Salmonellas

Most other serotypes of salmonella are pathogens of lower animals which are transmitted incidentally to man. Poultry and egg products account for about 50% of human cases; meats, dairy products, pet turtles and person-to-person spread within hospitals account for most of the remainder. Many cases of salmonellosis are sporadic, but large and small outbreaks traceable to a common source also occur frequently. In a typical instance, a food handler becomes infected through the handling of infected chicken carcasses. His hands then become contaminated from his faeces and small numbers of organisms are inoculated into food which he prepares. If this food is held at a temperature favourable for growth of salmonellas, the small inoculum of organisms may grow to a large population capable of producing infection in most individuals who eat the food. Similarly, batches of powdered egg products containing thousands of eggs may become contaminated through inclusion of a single heavily infected egg. There is now good evidence that intact chicken eggs may become contaminated with salmonellas. The large animal reservoir of salmonella species other than *S. typhi* has made it impossible to prevent a steady increase in the incidence of human salmonellosis during the past several decades.

Asymptomatic infection is extremely common. This is especially important in food handlers, who are both at high risk due to occupational exposure and responsible for transmission to others.

Infection with salmonella species other than *S. typhi* can cause several different clinical syndromes.
•*Enterocolitis*   Fever, nausea and vomiting, myalgia and headache followed by diarrhoea. Usually a self-limiting disease lasting 2–3 days.

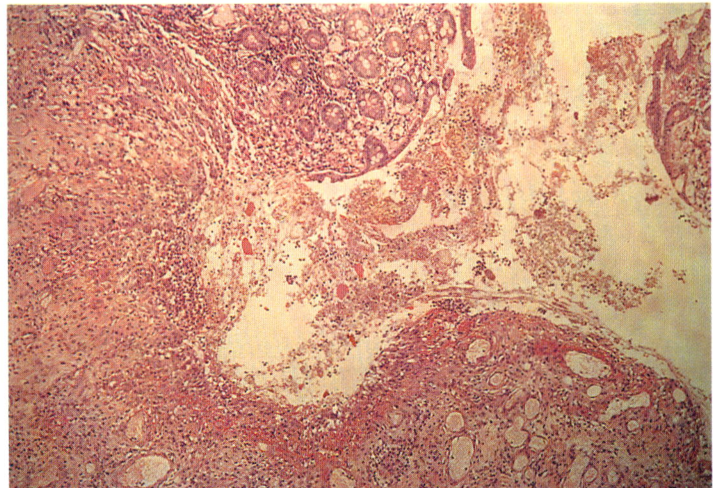

Fig. 2.32 Salmonellosis. Flask-shaped undermining ulcer with necrosis of the epithelium and extrusion of necrotic tissue, fibrin and mucus. By courtesy of Dr J. Newman.

•*Enteric fever* Similar to typhoid fever (fever, muscle aches and headache without diarrhoea) but usually milder and of shorter duration. Severe intestinal infection may produce histopathological changes similar to those seen in typhoid fever (Fig. 2.32).

•*Localized infection* Metastatic infection of vascular structures, bone and a wide variety of other tissues secondary to bacteraemia. This type of disease is especially common in infection due to *S. choleraesuis.*

•*Bacteraemia* Seen with recurrences following antibiotic therapy in patients with AIDS.

Faecal excretion of the organism for a few weeks following infection is very common, but persistent faecal excretion for more than a year after symptomatic or asymptomatic infection is rare (less than 1%) with organisms other than *S. typhi.*

Antimicrobial therapy is not indicated in the usual case of salmonella enterocolitis, which lasts only 2–3 days without treatment. Administration of bacteriostatic agents such as chloramphenicol may prolong the duration of faecal excretion of the organism or even exacerbate the diarrhoea. Enteric fever, localized infections and bacteraemia should be treated with antimicrobial agents. Chloramphenicol, ampicillin, amoxicillin, trimethoprim–sulphamethoxazole and ciprofloxacin have all been effective in the treatment of these more serious infections. Antibiotic resistance, including multiple resistance, is common in salmonellas and varies in different parts of the world, so therapy should be based upon determination of *in vitro* susceptibility of the infecting strain.

Bacteriological diagnosis of typhoid fever can be made by isolation of the organism from the blood during the first weeks of the illness in more than 80% of patients. Stool cultures are usually positive during the second, third and fourth weeks of the illness. In infections due to other species of *Salmonella,* the organism may be isolated from the stools in patients with enterocolitis or from the blood in patients with enteric fever or other types of bacteraemia. The organisms are lactose-negative and colonies may be differentiated from those of *E. coli* and other lactose-fermenting organisms on MacConkey agar and other selective media (Fig. 2.33). In metastatic abscesses or other types of localized infections the organisms can usually be readily isolated from specimens taken from the lesion.

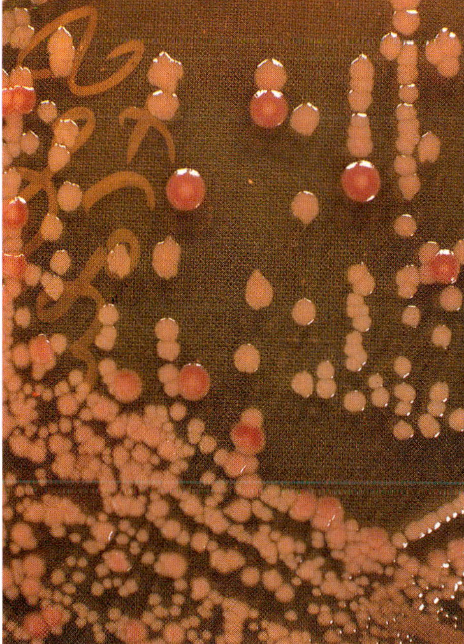

Fig. 2.33 Salmonellosis. Lactose-negative (light pink) colonies of salmonella growing on MacConkey agar, with a few lactose positive (deep pink) colonies of *E.coli.* By courtesy of Dr J. Hutchison.

CAMPYLOBACTER INFECTION

Campylobacters are motile, non-spore-forming, comma-shaped, gram-negative rods formerly included in the genus *Vibrio* (Fig. 2.34). The eleven species are mainly pathogens or commensals of a wide variety of mammals and birds. The most important human pathogen is *C. jejuni.*

Campylobacter infection is a worldwide zoonosis. These organisms inhabit the gastrointestinal tracts

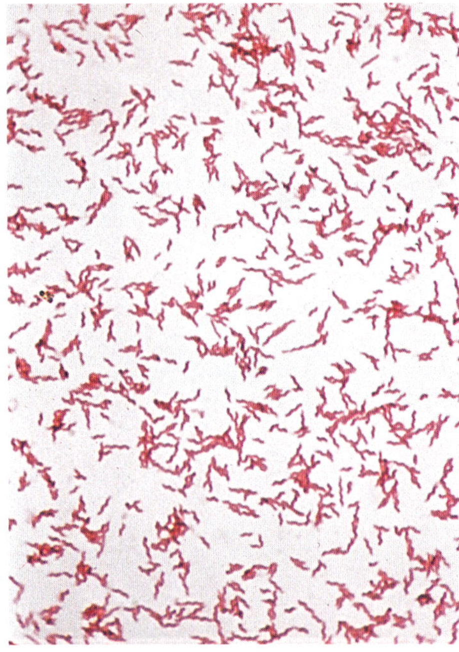

Fig. 2.34 *Campylobacter jejuni* infection. Gram stain showing gram-negative, comma-shaped bacilli of *C. jejuni*. By courtesy of Dr I. Farrell.

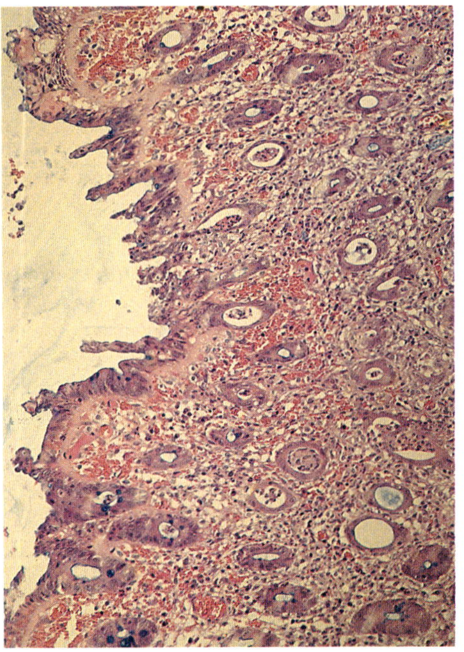

Fig. 2.35 *Campylobacter jejuni* infection. Inflammatory enteritis involving the entire mucosa with flattened, atrophic villi, necrotic debris in the lumina of the crypts and thickening of the basement membrane. Cresyl-fast violet stain. By courtesy of Dr J. Newman.

of many wild and domestic mammals and fowl. Intestinal carriage following initial infection in these animals may be lifelong; this vast animal reservoir is the source of most human infections. Humans acquire the organism by ingesting contaminated food (especially undercooked meat), water or unpasteurized milk. Less common routes of infection are through direct contact with infected pets, occupational exposure to farm animals or person-to-person transmission. Asymptomatic infection in food handlers is uncommon, in contrast to the situation with salmonellosis. In industrialized countries this infection is probably more common than salmonellosis or shigellosis. The prevalence of asymptomatic infection is very low. In developing countries up to 40% of children under 2 years may be infected and the organism is an important cause of diarrhoea in travellers to these countries.

The infective dose for campylobacters is similar to that for salmonellas, significantly higher than the minimum infective dose for shigellas. There may be a prodrome of fever, malaise, headache and myalgias for up to a day prior to onset of abdominal pain and diarrhoea, which may be mild or severe. Unless the proper microbiological studies are done the disease may be misdiagnosed as ulcerative colitis or Crohn's disease. *C. jejuni*, like the *Yersinia* species, may produce a pseudo-appendicitis

syndrome of terminal ileitis and mesenteric adenitis. Untreated patients usually excrete the organisms for 2–3 weeks after recovery. Antibiotic treatment results in rapid elimination of campylobacter organisms from the faeces, unlike the case in salmonellosis.

Histopathological examination reveals a diffuse, haemorrhagic, oedematous and exudative enteritis often accompanied by a non-specific colitis (Fig. 2.35). Although the organisms invade the intestinal mucosa in both man and lower animals, bacteraemia is rare (less than 1%) in human infections. Both enterotoxins and cytotoxins are produced by *C. jejuni*, but their significance in the pathogenesis of the infection is unknown.

C. fetus is also an important cause of human infections. Diarrhoeal disease is less common with this species, which more often produces systemic infection with bacteraemia and a wide variety of localized infections, especially in patients in whom the immune system is impaired. The organism seems to have a special ability to produce vascular infections such as endocarditis, mycotic aneurysm and thrombophlebitis.

A diagnosis of campylobacter infection is suspected on finding the comma-shaped, S-shaped or spiral organisms in a stool specimen stained with Gram or carbol-fuchsin stains (Fig. 2.36)

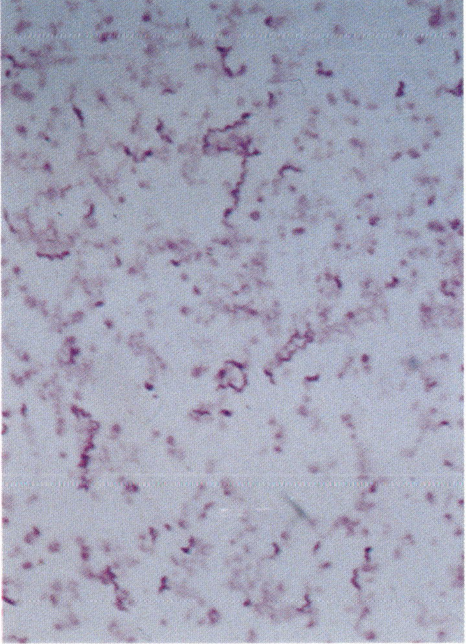

Fig. 2.36 Organisms of the genus *Campylobacter* are now recognized as an important cause of gastroenteritis. They are gram-negative rods; many are curved or show a 'seagull' configuration.

Microbiological diagnosis is confirmed by isolating the organism from either stools or blood, depending upon the type of infection. These organisms are microaerophilic, growing best in an atmosphere of 5–10% oxygen. Incubation at 42°C, the addition of cephalothin to the medium or passage of the specimen through a 0.65 mm filter may facilitate isolation of campylobacter from faecal specimens.

Most patients with diarrhoeal disease due to campylobacters can be treated effectively with replacement of fluid and electrolyte losses, without antibiotic therapy. As with salmonellosis, no clinical benefit can be demonstrated in the treatment of mild cases of diarrhoeal disease. Antimicrobial therapy should be used in the patient who has high fever, bloody diarrhoea or more than 8 stools per day, in the patient who is getting worse or has not begun to improve by the time the diagnosis is made, and in the patient who remains symptomatic for longer than a week. Erythromycin appears to be beneficial in the treatment of severe illness. Campylobacters are extremely susceptible to the newer fluoroquinolone agents *in vitro,* and limited experience indicates that these agents are effective in the treatment of campylobacter infections. Campylobacters are resistant to the penicillins and to trimethoprim–sulphamethoxazole.

YERSINIA INFECTIONS

Yersinia enterocolitica

Y. enterocolitica is a widely distributed pathogen of animals which causes diarrhoea in humans primarily in cooler climates. In some northern European countries, Canada and Australia, *Y. enterocolitica* is more common than *Shigella* and rivals *Salmonella* and *Campylobacter* as a cause of enteric disease. It has been isolated from a wide variety of mammals, birds, fish and invertebrates, and also from lakes, streams, well water and vegetables. Most human infections follow ingestion of contaminated food (especially raw pork), water or milk. Person-to-person transmission is uncommon, but nosocomial spread has occurred. Serotypes 0:3, 0:8 and 0:9 are the most virulent and cause most cases of bacteraemic infection. Isolates from the inanimate environment usually belong to other, non-virulent serotypes. Virulence is associated with plasmids which code for certain specific outer membrane proteins.

The incubation period is 1–10 days. The illness usually lasts 1–2 weeks, but the organism may be found in the stool for several weeks after clinical recovery. In children under the age of 5 years, the

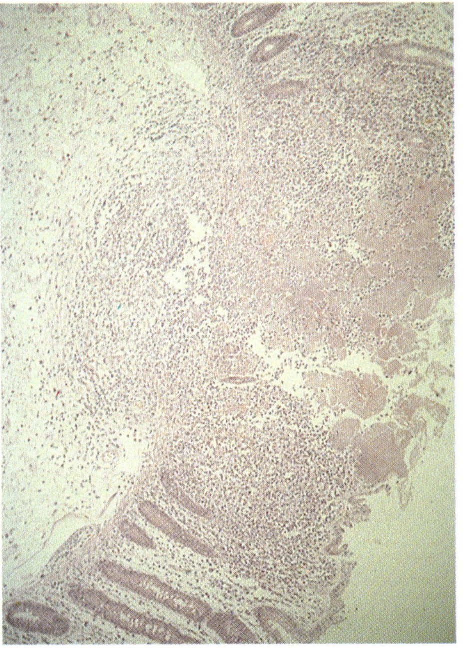

Fig. 2.37 Yersinia infection. Necrosis and ulceration of intestinal mucosa overlying a hyperplastic lymphoid follicle. The inflammatory infiltrate is composed primarily of mononuclear cells. By courtesy of Dr J. Newman.

most common type of illness is enterocolitis, characterized by diarrhoea, low-grade fever and abdominal pain. White and red blood cells are found in the stools, which are sometimes grossly bloody.

Most of these infections are self-limited and serious complications are uncommon.

In older children terminal ileitis (Figs 2.37, 2.38 & 2.39) and mesenteric adenitis (Figs 2.40 & 2.41)

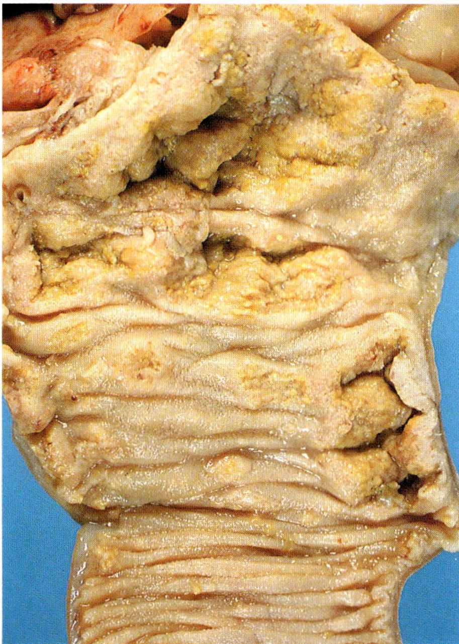

Fig. 2.38 Yersinia infection. Gross specimen of ileum, showing superficial necrosis of the intestinal mucosa with several well-defined deep and superficial ulcers. By courtesy of Dr J. Newman.

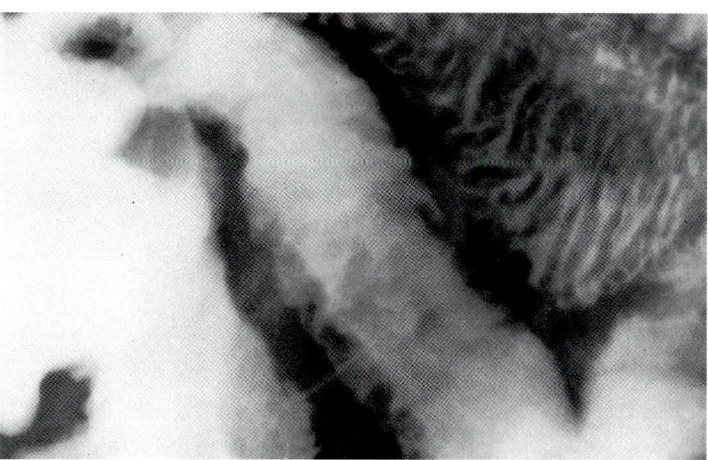

Fig. 2.39 Barium study in a patient with yersinia ileitis showing nodularity and shallow ulceration in the distal ileum.

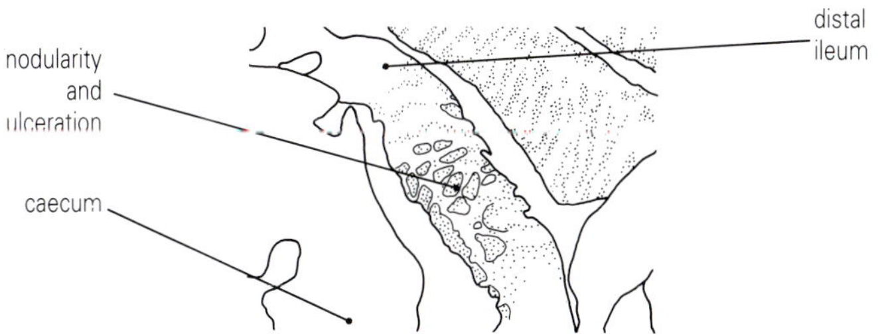

are most common. Most patients exhibit fever, leucocytosis, abdominal pain and tenderness in the right lower quadrant. Nausea, vomiting and diarrhoea are present in a minority. The clinical picture may be indistinguishable from acute appendicitis and appendectomy has been performed in many patients. Physical examination may reveal a tender, sausage-shaped mass in the right lower quadrant. Ultrasonography is valuable in distinguishing between the terminal ileitis/mesenteric adenitis syndrome and appendicitis. In these patients the appendix is normal or only slightly inflamed, but the wall of the terminal ileum is grossly thickened with mucosal ulcerations and involvement of Peyer's patches and, on microscopic examination, exhibits inflammation and oedema (see Figs 2.37 & 2.38). *Y. enterocolitica* can be cultured from the tissue of the terminal ileum and from involved lymph nodes.

Bacteraemia and focal extraintestinal infections are seen primarily in older adults. Focal infections include pharyngitis, cellulitis and localized abscesses in various organs. Cirrhosis and haemochromatosis are associated with an increased incidence of bacteraemia due to this organism. Reactive polyarthritis and erythema nodosum also occur most commonly in older patients.

Diagnosis is best made by isolating the organisms, which are lactose-negative, on MacConkey agar. Since *Y. enterocolitica* multiplies at cold temperatures, isolation from stool specimens can be facilitated by cold-enrichment techniques.

Agglutinating antibodies appear during the first week and reach a peak in the second week of illness. Cross-reactions occur between antigens of *Y. enterocolitica* and those of *Brucella abortus*, rickettsias, salmonellas and thyroid tissue.

The organism is sensitive to trimethoprim–sulphamethoxazole, aminoglycosides, tetracyclines, third-generation cephalosporins and fluoroquinolones. It is resistant to most penicillins and first-generation cephalosporins. Treatment with antibiotics is not required in cases of enterocolitis or the terminal ileitis/mesenteric adenitis syndrome, but more invasive types of infection such as bacteraemia and focal abscesses should be treated.

Yersinia pseudotuberculosis

Yersinia pseudotuberculosis is primarily a pathogen of wild and domestic mammals and birds around the world. Human infection is uncommon and occurs primarily in individuals who have contact with infected domestic animals. The illness produced in man by *Y. pseudotuberculosis* resembles that resulting from *Y. enterocolitica*. Most patients have an appendicitis-like syndrome with fever and pain in the right lower quadrant of the abdomen, caused by terminal ileitis and mesenteric adenitis. A few patients with sepsis and bacteraemia have been reported. *Y. pseudotuberculosis* is more antibiotic-sensitive than *Y. enterocolitica*; otherwise the recommended treatment for the two types of infection is the same.

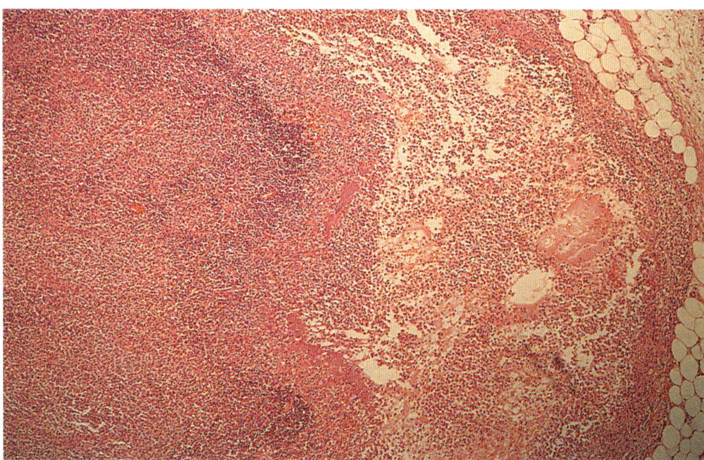

Fig. 2.40 Yersinia infection. Hyperplasia and inflammatory infiltration of a mesenteric lymph node. By courtesy of Dr C. Edwards.

CLOSTRIDIUM INFECTIONS

Clostridium perfringens

Clostridium perfringens type A is a very common cause of food poisoning, and *C. perfringens* type C causes a much more serious necrotizing enteritis in various parts of the world. *C. perfringens* food poisoning is due to a heat-labile enterotoxin released during germination of spores in the food or in the gastrointestinal tract after ingestion. The clinical picture consists of diarrhoea and abdominal cramps, usually without fever or vomiting. Outbreaks usually follow ingestion of meats and gravies. The classic vehicle is a meat pie with a crust: the vegetative cells but not the spores are killed during cooking; the crust maintains anaerobic conditions while the spores germinate; and the bacteria release toxin as the pie cools. Necrotizing enteritis is most often associated with invasion of the bowel wall by *C. perfringens* type C and may be due to the action of the β-toxin, which is a potent lecithinase that causes cell lysis (Fig. 2.42). Sporadic cases are seen around the world, in adults and especially in children. Epidemics have been described in northern Germany (Darmbrand) in the mid-1940s, and in the highlands of New Guinea during ritual orgiastic feasting on inadequately cooked pork (*pig-bel*). The illness begins suddenly with severe abdominal pain, vomiting, bloody diarrhoea, prostration and shock. Pathological findings include acute patchy necrotizing lesions (Fig. 2.43), which may progress rapidly to segmental gangrene with gas in the mucosa, mesentery or regional lymph nodes. Gas may be seen radiographically in the wall of the small bowel. Treatment includes supportive care with replacement of food and electrolyte losses and decompression of the bowel. Penicillin G should be given intravenously in large doses and *C. perfringens* type C antiserum containing β-antitoxin should be administered if available. Complications of paralyt-

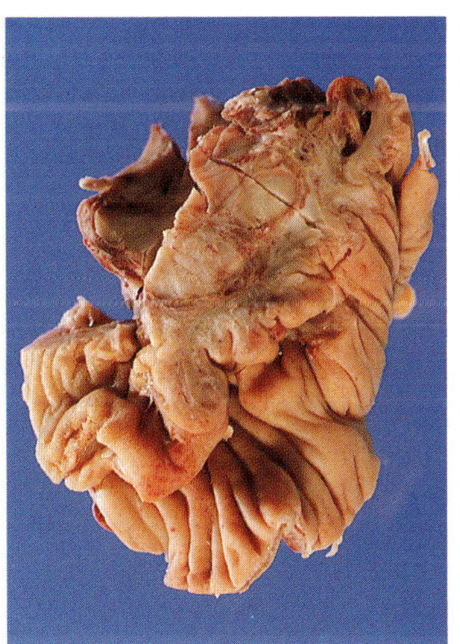
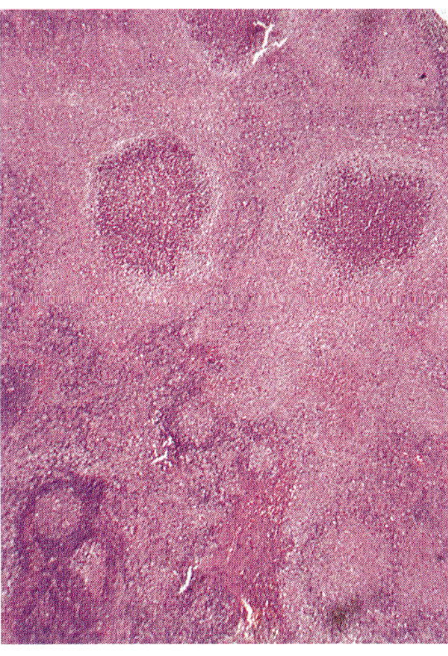

Fig. 2.41 Yersiniosis. Left: Resected ileum showing two enlarged fleshy nodes in the mesentery and some overlying mucosal granularity. The nodes contained the classical necrotic inflammatory foci. Right: The basic nodal architecture is preserved in yersiniosis but many of the follicular germinal centers are replaced with polymorphs with some necrosis from tiny micro-abscesses. ×10. H&E stain.

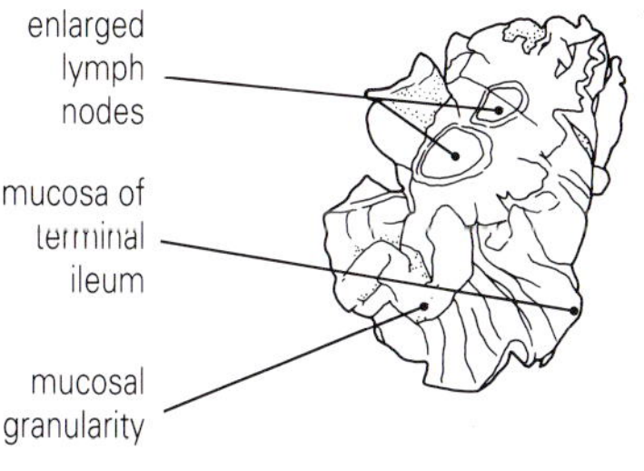

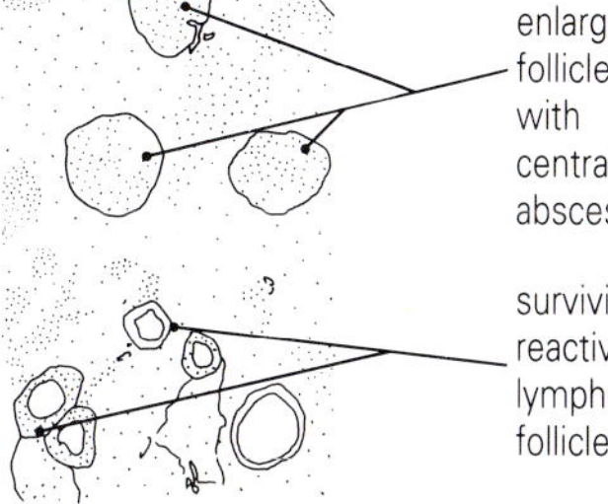

ic ileus, strangulation and perforation of the bowel may necessitate abdominal exploration and resection of involved segments of the intestine.

Clostridium difficile (Antibiotic-associated colitis)

Many patients develop mild, transient diarrhoea during or following antibiotic therapy, probably due to alterations in the normal flora of the intestine. A more serious antibiotic-associated colitis (AAC), which may progress to full-blown pseudomembranous colitis, is associated with the presence of *Clostridium difficile* and its cytotoxins. This organism is present in the intestinal tract in approximately 3% of normal adults. The prevalence may be much higher in some populations,

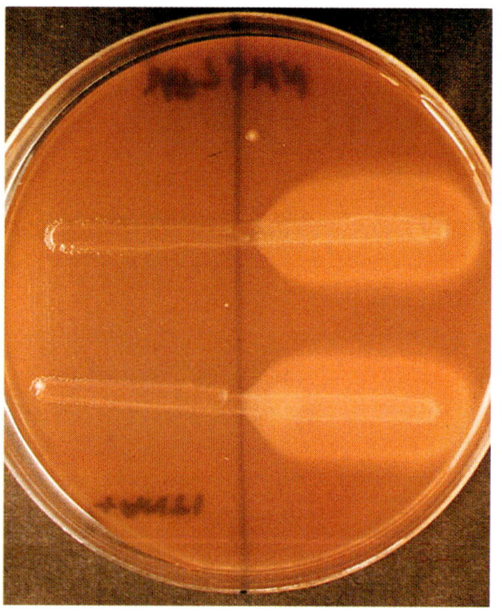

Fig. 2.42 *Clostridium welchii (perfringens)*. Nagler's reaction detects the lecithinase produced by *C. welchii* which gives a precipitate in egg yolk media. There are two parallel streams of growth. Zones of opacity are seen on the right half but not on the left, on which antitoxin was placed before inoculation.

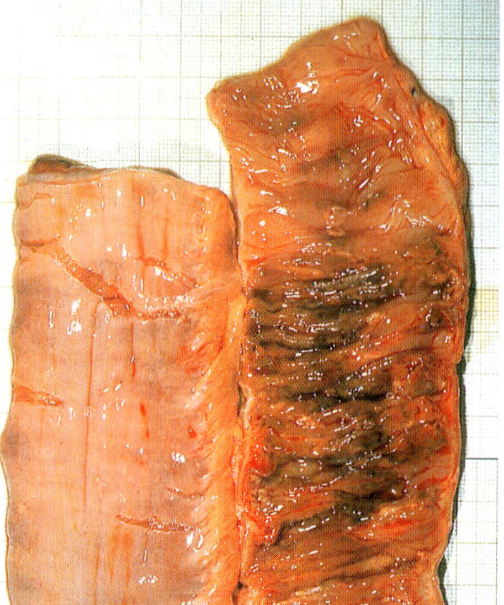

Fig. 2.43 Necrotizing enteritis (*pig-bel*). Gross specimen of small bowel from a case seen in Uganda. The lower piece of opened jejunum shows the greyish-black areas of necrosis, particularly involving the superficial part of the transverse mucosal folds. By courtesy of Professor M. S. R. Hutt.

especially in hospitalized patients who are elderly or debilitated or who have recently undergone abdominal surgery. AAC may follow treatment with a wide variety of antimicrobial agents, most commonly ampicillin, clindamycin and cephalosporins, but also including tetracyclines, erythromycin, trimethoprim–sulphamethoxazole and even metronidazole, which is used in the treatment of this disease. The incidence varies widely from one geographical area to the next; the presence of clusters of cases strongly suggests person-to-person spread of the organism. The spores are resistant to many environmental influences and can persist for long periods on the hands of hospital personnel. Most strains of *C. difficile* isolated from patients with AAC produce toxins A and B; the colitis apparently results from production of toxin in the intestinal lumen. Approximately 90% of adult patients with antibiotic-associated diarrhoea who have either *C. difficile* or its toxins demonstrated in the faeces have either gross or microscopic evidence of colitis. On the other hand, up to 50% of newborn infants may be colonized at least transiently with *C. difficile*; these infants remain well in spite of the presence of large amounts of toxin in the bowel.

The role of antibiotic therapy in precipitating AAC is not fully understood. These agents may suppress the normal bacterial flora, allowing overgrowth of *C. difficile* (Fig. 2.44), or they may stimulate production of toxins by this organism. A similar if not identical disease was observed in the pre-antibiotic era, and not all patients who develop pseudomembranous colitis at the present time have received antibiotics.

The disease usually begins 4–10 days after initiation of antibiotic therapy with the explosive onset of profuse, watery or mucoid, green, foul smelling diarrhoea. In about one-third of patients diarrhoea begins after discontinuation of antibiotics, usually within a few days but occasionally up to 6 weeks after therapy has been stopped. Crampy abdominal pain, abdominal tenderness, fever up to 41°C and leucocytosis are commonly present. Approximately half have leucocytes present in the diarrhoeal stools. Signs of acute surgical abdomen, toxic megacolon, perforation of the colon and peritonitis occur in a few patients. The case fatality rate is 10–20% in untreated cases.

The diagnosis is made by demonstrating colitis in association with *C. difficile* and/or its toxins. The characteristic plaques of pseudomembranous colitis are yellowish white, 1–5 mm in diameter, with an erythematous border or base (Figs 2.45 & 2.46). They may occur anywhere in the colon, but are

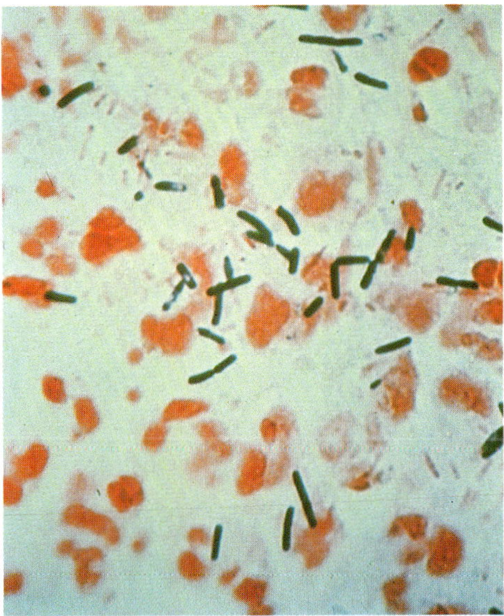

Fig. 2.44 Antibiotic-associated colitis. Gram stain of faeces showing large gram-positive spore-forming rod-shaped cells of *C. difficile*, along with small numbers of gram-negative organisms and many inflammatory cells. By courtesy of Dr R. Fekety.

most common in the rectosigmoid region where they are readily seen on sigmoidoscopy (Figs 2.47, 2.48 & 2.49). Irregularity of the mucosal outline may be seen on plain x-ray films of the abdomen or on barium enema examination (Fig. 2.50). In a few cases plaques occur only in the proximal colon and colonoscopy is required to visualize them. On microscopic examination they are found to be com-

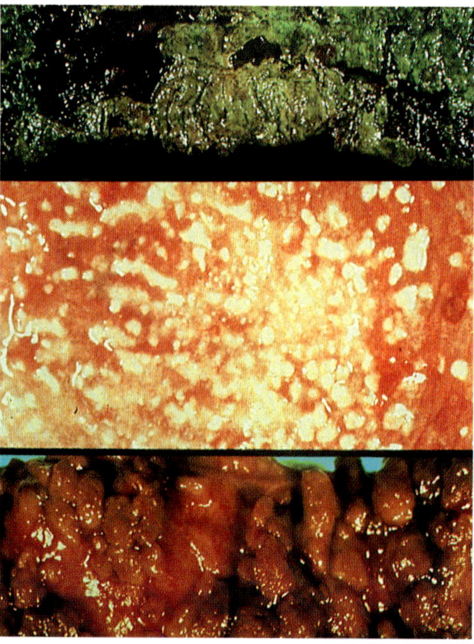

Fig. 2.45 Gross specimens of colons from fatal cases of antibiotic-associated colitis. Top: Extensive inflammatory pseudomembrane. Middle: numerous small plaques, some almost confluent. Bottom: Confluent pseudomembrane covering most of the epithelial surface. By courtesy of Dr F. Pittman (top) and Dr R. Fekety (middle and bottom).

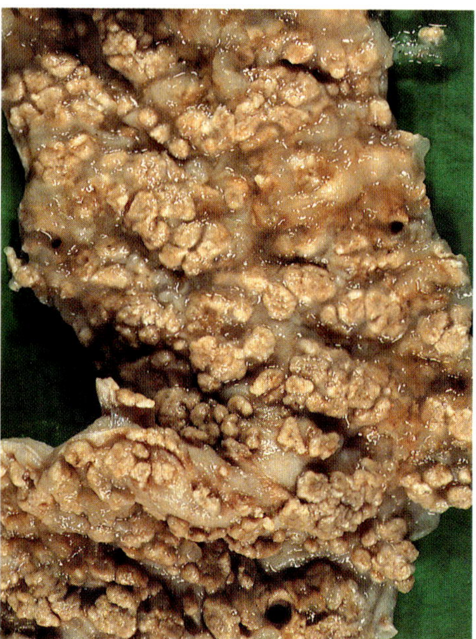

Fig. 2.46 Macroscopic appearance of typical pseudomembranous colitis showing the discrete yellow plaques.

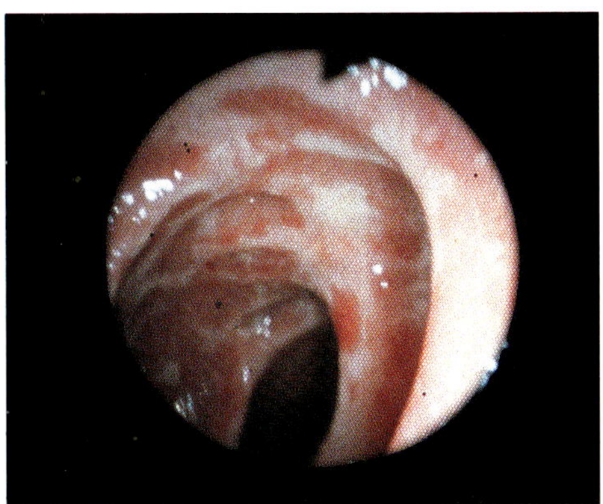

Fig. 2.47 Sigmoidoscopic view of pseudomembranous colitis due to antibiotic treatment. The yellow-white 'membrane' contrasts with the reddened colonic mucosa. By courtesy of Prof. R. Hunt.

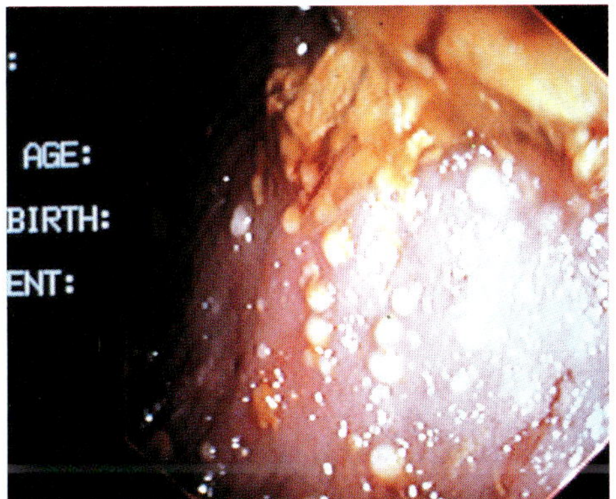

Fig. 2.48 Antibiotic-associated colitis. Sigmoidoscopic view demonstrating multiple pseudomembranous lesions in a patient with antibiotic-associated colitis due to *Clostridium difficile*. By courtesy of Dr J. Cunningham.

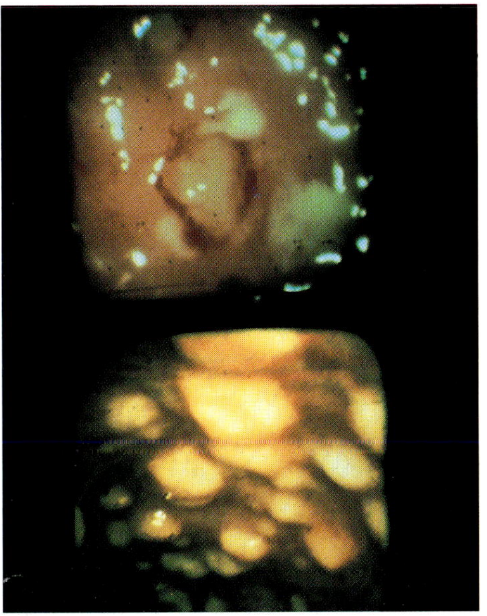

Fig. 2.49 Colonoscopic views of antibiotic-associated colitis. Top: Several whitish or yellowish plaques surrounded by haemorrhagic borders. Bottom: Numerous characteristic whitish plaques. By courtesy of Dr F. Pittman (top) and Dr R. Fekety (bottom).

posed of fibrin, mucus, necrotic epithelial cells and leucocytes (Fig. 2.51). In less severe cases only a diffuse microscopic colitis without plaque formation is present. *C. difficile* is readily isolated from most cases of AAC by culturing stool specimens anaerobically at 35–37°C on selective media. *C. difficile* toxin B may be detected with assays employing monolayers of fibroblasts or other cell lines (Fig. 2.52). Most patients with AAC due to *C. difficile* have large amounts of toxin in their stool filtrates. Neutralization of the cytopathic effects by appropriate antiserum establishes the identity of the toxin.

If the patient has only mild diarrhoea, treatment should consist only of discontinuation of the antibiotic and replacement of fluid and electrolyte losses.

If the diarrhoea is severe and/or systemic illness is present, or if the patient fails to improve within 48 hours on supportive therapy, antimicrobial therapy should be initiated. The most effective agent is vancomycin, given orally. Treatment should be continued for 5–7 days, or until toxin disappears from the stools. In less severe cases, metronidazole may be given. This drug is much less expensive than vancomycin. Limited experience indicates that bacitracin is also effective in the treatment of this disease. Recurrences develop in 10–20% of patients. These should be treated with vancomycin, regardless of which drug was used for initial treatment. Use of opiates and other antimotility agents should be avoided.

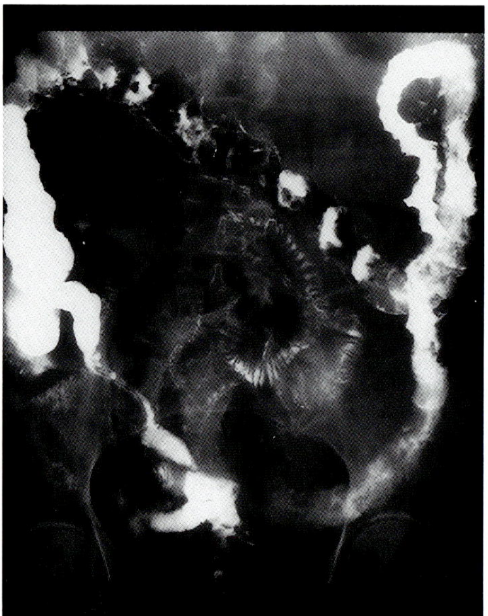

Fig. 2.50 Antibiotic-associated colitis. Barium follow-through showing narrowing of the lumen of the colon, thickened haustral folds ('thumbprinting') and numerous small mucosal ulcerations. By courtesy of Dr R. Noble.

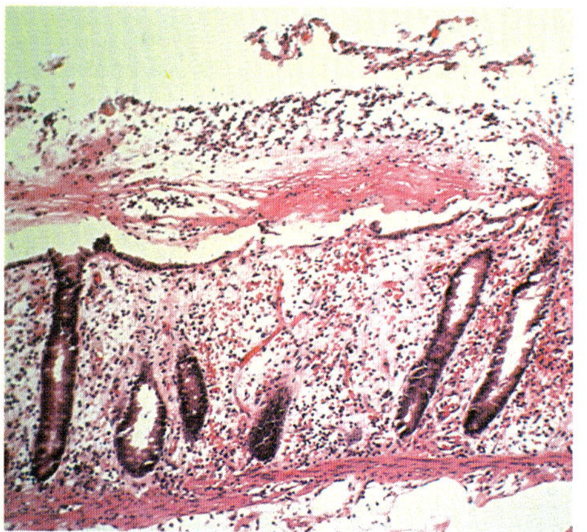

Fig. 2.51 Antibiotic-associated colitis. A section of colon showing intense inflammatory response with the characteristic 'plaque'. H&E stain.

RECTAL SPIROCHAETOSIS

Rectal spirochaetosis is a poorly understood condition seen in approximately 36% of homosexual men and less commonly in heterosexual individuals. It is sometimes associated with chronic diarrhoea. The numerous organisms often form a superficial haematoxyphilic layer covering the epithelium (Figs 2.53 & 2.54).

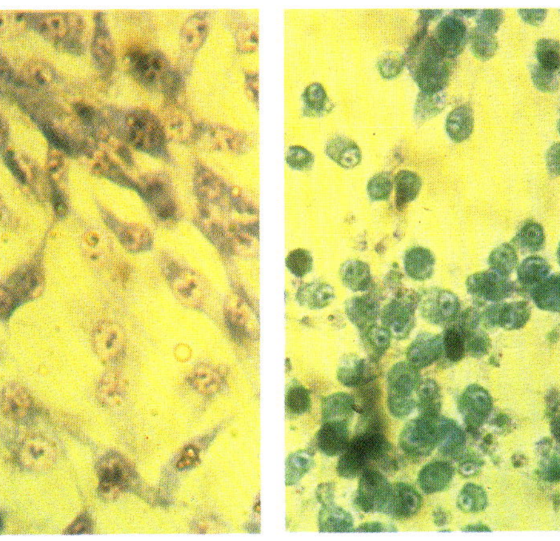

Fig. 2.52 Antibiotic-associated colitis. Assay for *Clostridium difficile* toxin showing normal baby hamster kidney cells (left) and cells after exposure to toxin (right). Note the rounding up of cells following exposure to toxin. By courtesy of Dr R. Fekety.

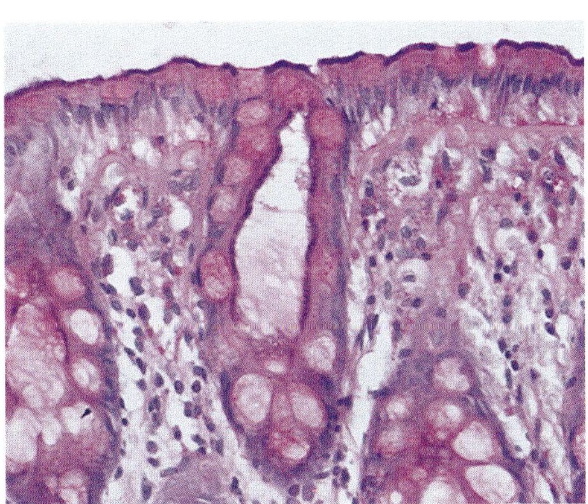

Fig. 2.53 Rectal spirochaetosis. The numerous organisms form a superficial PAS-positive layer over the epithelium. There is also superficial oedema between the basal cell layer and the distorted basement membrane and lymphocytic infiltration of the lamina propria. By courtesy of Dr J. Newman.

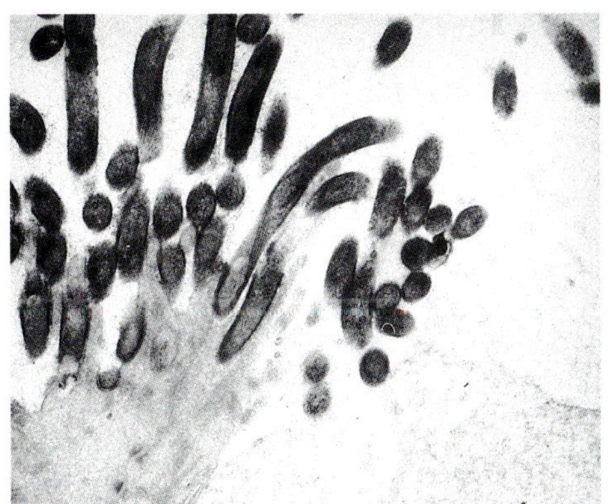

Fig. 2.54 Rectal spirochaetosis. Electron micrograph showing numerous organisms attached to the epithelial surface of the intestinal mucosa. By courtesy of Dr J. Newman.

TUBERCULOUS ENTERITIS

Infection of the gastrointestinal tract by the tubercle bacillus may be either primary or secondary to pulmonary or miliary tuberculosis. Prior to widespread pasteurization of milk, intestinal tuberculosis was often caused by *Mycobacterium bovis*; now in industrialized countries nearly all cases are caused by *M. tuberculosis*. The ileocaecal area is involved most often (Figs 2.55 & 2.56), although extensive involvement of the small bowel and colon may also be seen (Figs 2.57 & 2.58). The most common clinical features are fever, abdominal pain, weight loss and diarrhoea, sometimes with

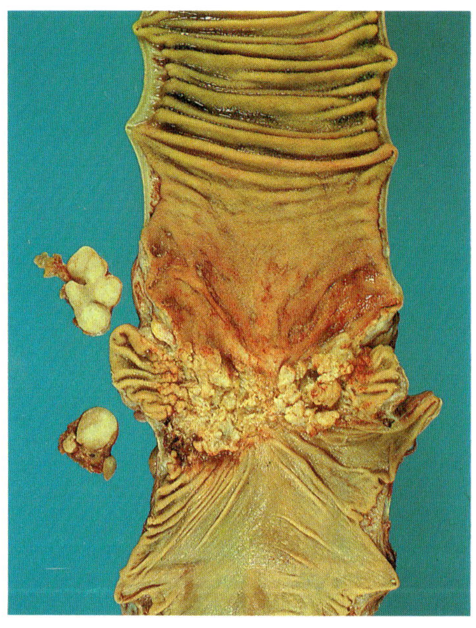

Fig. 2.55 Tuberculous enteritis. Transverse ulceration and caseous necrosis involving the intestinal wall and adjacent lymph nodes. By courtesy of Dr J. Newman.

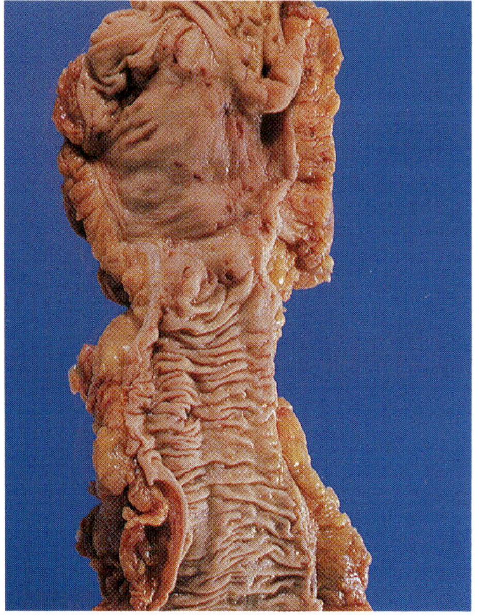

Fig. 2.56 Macroscopic appearance of the ileocaecal region in intestinal tuberculosis, showing the thickened, flattened, featureless caecal mucosa and small haemorrhagic ulcers.

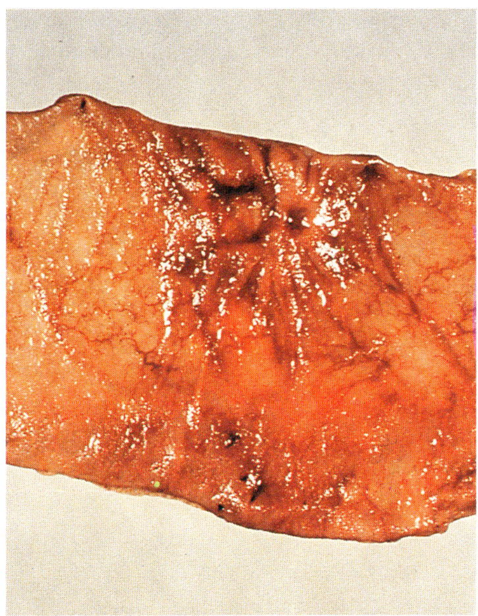

Fig. 2.57 Tuberculosis enteritis. Autopsy specimen of colon showing an oval ulcer. The bowel wall is generally somewhat thickened.

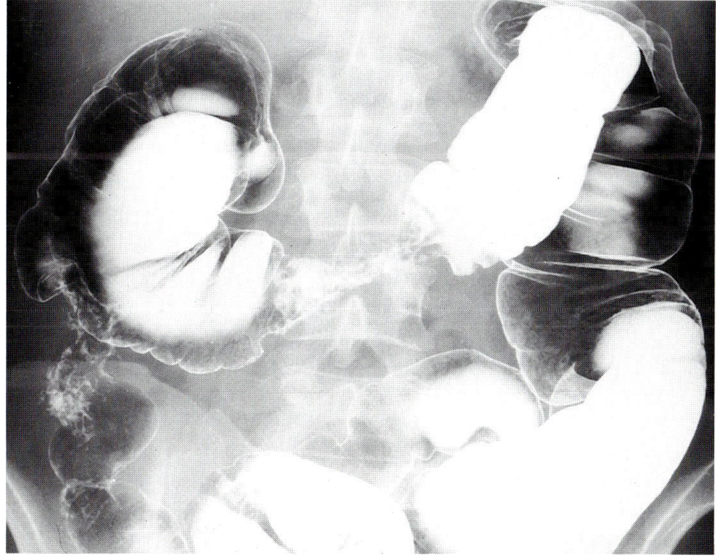

Fig. 2.58 Barium enema showing tuberculous stricturing in the transverse colon and ascending colon.

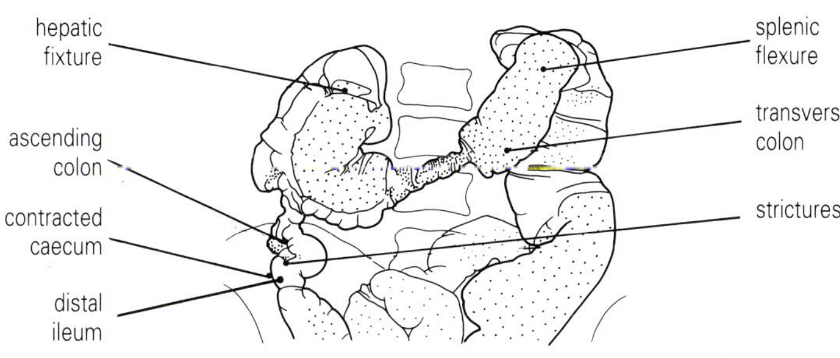

a fixed palpable mass in the ileocaecal area. Obstruction, haemorrhage and malabsorption are occasional complications. On barium studies and even at surgery the hypertrophic or ulcerative lesions may be difficult to distinguish from carcinoma or Crohn's disease (Fig. 2.59). Other diseases

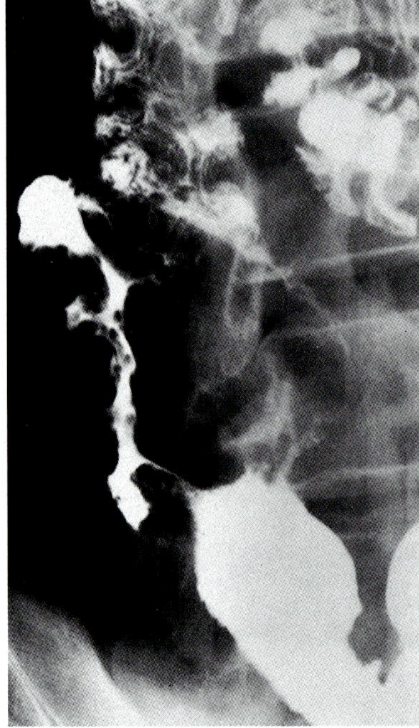

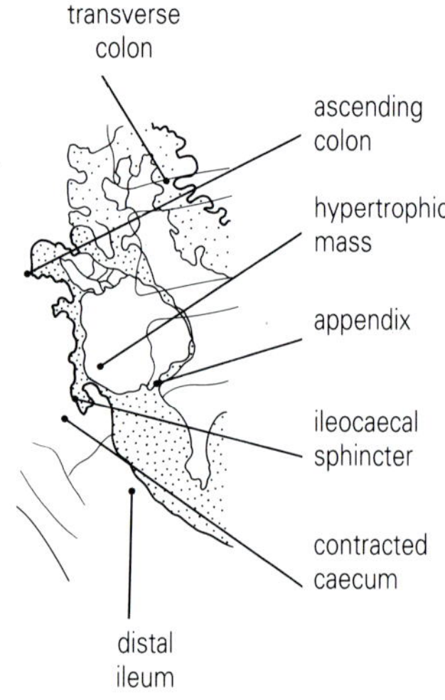

Fig. 2.59 Barium enema in hypertrophic TB, mainly affecting the ascending colon in a 32-year-old Indian presenting with a large mass in the right iliac fossa.

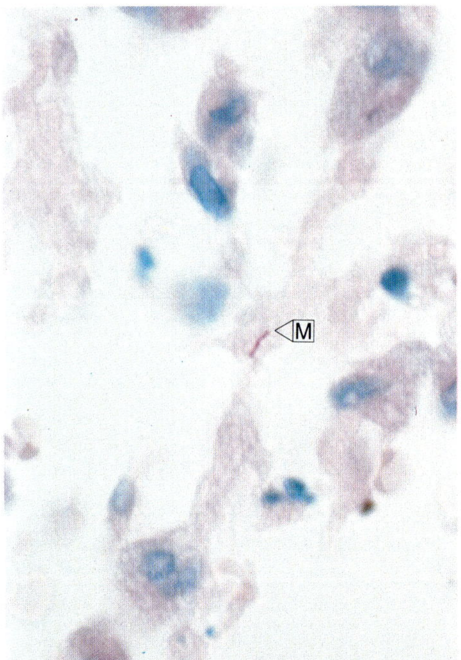

Fig. 2.60 An acid-fast mycobacterium (M). ×1200. Ziehl-Neelsen stain.

which may resemble intestinal tuberculosis are sarcoidosis, actinomycosis, amoeboma and periappendiceal abscess. Definitive diagnosis often requires demonstration of acid-fast bacilli in the tissue by stain or culture (Fig. 2.60). Caseation necrosis is often absent from the intestinal lesion but may be seen in the mesenteric nodes (Figs 2.61 & 2.62). Treatment is the same as for other forms of extrapulmonary tuberculosis.

MYCOBACTERIUM AVIUM–INTRACELLULARE

Approximately 50% of AIDS patients who have disseminated infection with *Mycobacterium avium–intracellulare* (MAI) have involvement of the intestine. These patients have, in addition to the fever, malaise and weight loss exhibited by all patients with disseminated MAI infection, chronic diar-

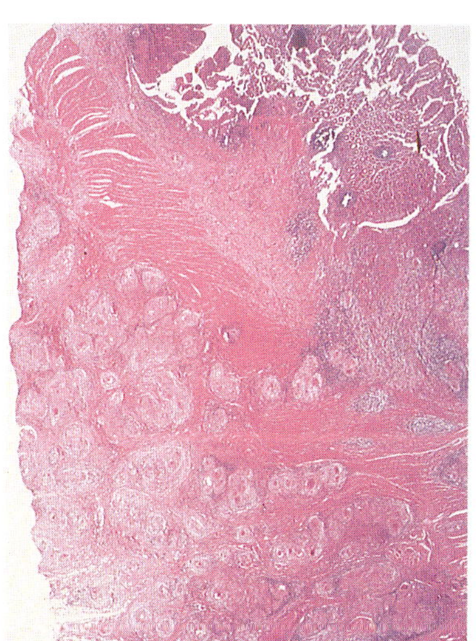

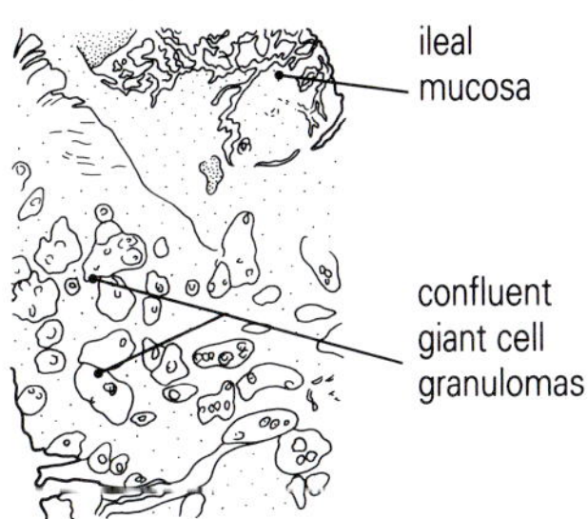

Fig. 2.61 Confluent giant cell granulomas penetrating the full thickness of the intestinal wall in tuberculosis. By contrast, in Crohn's disease the granulomas are smaller and usually solitary. ×10. H&E stain.

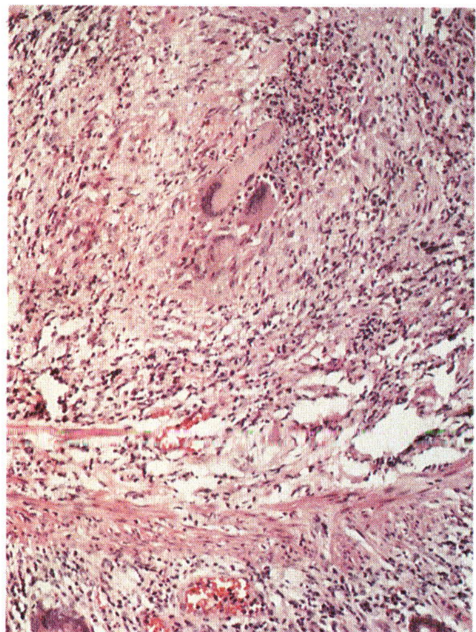

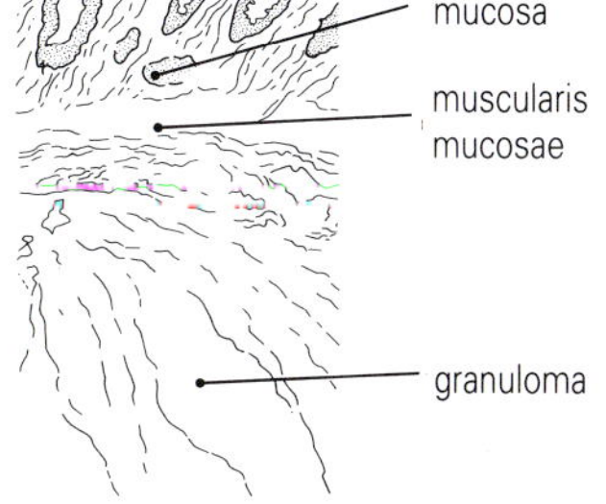

Fig. 2.62 Tuberculous enteritis. Histological section of colon showing a granuloma with lymphocytes, epithelioid cells and giant cells, but without caseation, in the submucosa. H&E stain.

rhoea and abdominal pain. Like other patients with disseminated MAI infection, they have persistent bacteraemia, but also have positive stool cultures for this organism. Histopathological studies of the gut typically show absent or poorly formed granulomas and acid-fast bacilli within macrophages (Fig. 2.63). There are two clinical syndromes, which may overlap: chronic diarrhoea and abdominal pain in patients with invasion of the colon; and chronic malabsorption and steatorrhoea with Whipple's disease-like histopathological changes in the small bowel (Fig. 2.64). The latter patients have large numbers of mycobacteria within macrophages in the lamina propria of the small intestine and enlarged mesenteric lymph nodes infiltrated with acid-fast bacteria (Fig. 2.65).

Most isolates of MAI are susceptible to ansamycin (rifabutine), clofazimine, cycloserine, ethambutol and ethionamide, but are resistant to isoniazid and rifampin. New macrolide antibiotics, including azithromycin and clarithromycin, appear promising. However, treatment with even the most active agents has not been highly effective. Modest improvement in the clinical symptoms and reduction in the intensity of the bacteraemia is about all that can be accomplished with present therapy.

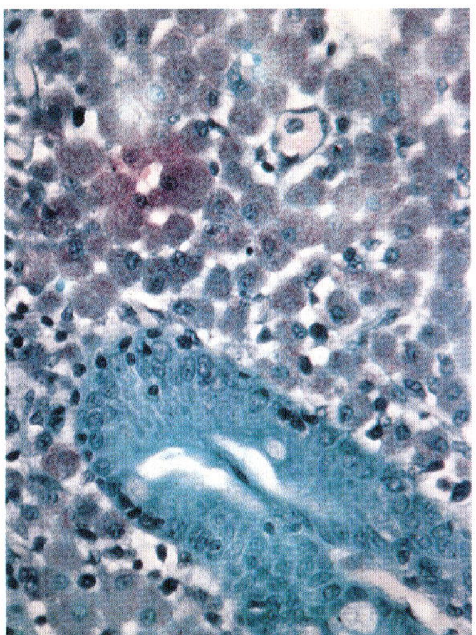

Fig. 2.63 Enteritis due to *Mycobacterium avium–intracellulare*. FITE stain showing acid-fast organisms (red) and intense chronic inflammatory response without granuloma formation in a patient with AIDS. By courtesy of Dr M. B. Cohen.

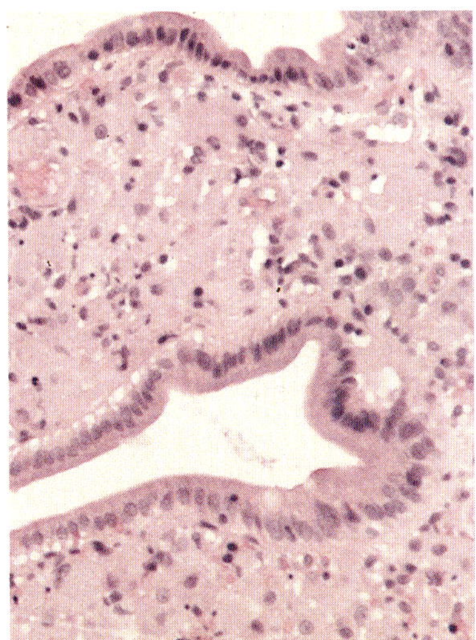

Fig. 2.64 Enteritis due to *Mycobacterium avium–intracellulare*. Section of small intestine from a patient with AIDS with a Whipple's disease-like syndrome, showing many foam-filled macrophages in the lamina propria. By courtesy of Dr R. S. Markin.

TROPICAL SPRUE

Tropical sprue is an inflammatory disease of the small bowel mucosa with many features which suggest that it is an infectious disease. The geographical distribution includes the Caribbean area, northern South America, tropical and southern Africa, India, and southeast Asia (Fig. 2.66). It occurs in both natives and expatriates from temperate regions, usually after one or two years residence in the tropics. Both sporadic and epidemic outbreaks are seen.

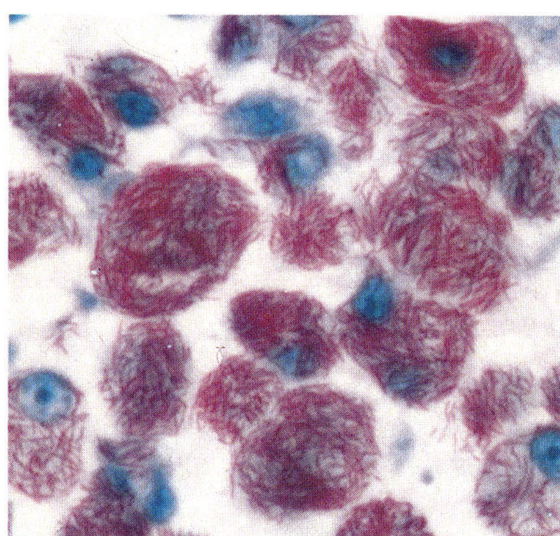

Fig. 2.65 Enteritis due to *Mycobacterium avium–intracellulare*. Acid-fast stain of a section of small intestine in a patient with AIDS, showing abundant acid-fast bacilli in macrophages. By courtesy of Dr R. S. Markin.

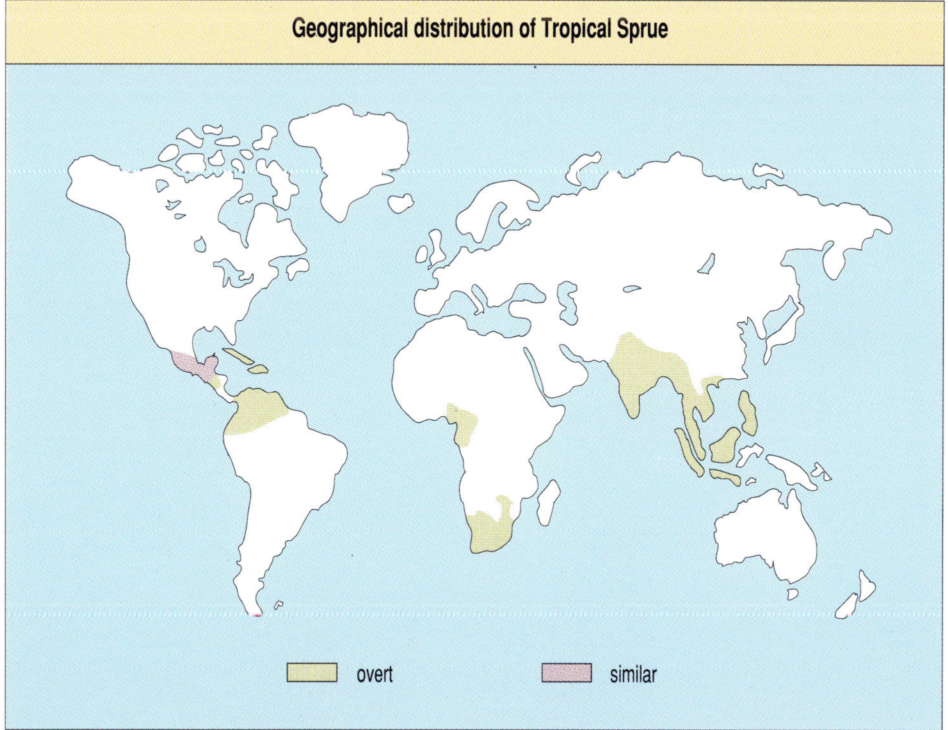

Fig. 2.66 Map showing the distribution of tropical sprue and disorders resembling sprue.

Onset, at least in expatriates, is often acute with explosive diarrhoea accompanied by fever, malaise, weakness and nausea; this is followed by chronic diarrhoea, abdominal distension and crampy abdominal pain. Examination of fluid from the upper small intestine reveals contamination by coliform bacteria, most commonly *Klebsiella pneumoniae*, with *E. coli* or *Enterobacter cloacae* found less frequently. Most bacterial strains isolated from patients produce heat-labile and heat-stable enterotoxins which differ from the LT and ST toxins of *E. coli*. Many of the strains also produce ethanol, which may damage the intestinal mucosa. Tropical sprue may be a consequence of chronic contamination of the small intestine by toxigenic coliform bacteria following an initial episode of acute bacterial enteritis.

Eventually symptoms of folate deficiency develop, including glossitis, anaemia and weight loss. There is net secretion of water and electrolytes in the small bowel and malabsorption of carbohydrate, amino acids, fats and vitamins.

Definitive diagnosis is made by examination of the stools, to exclude giardia and other parasites,

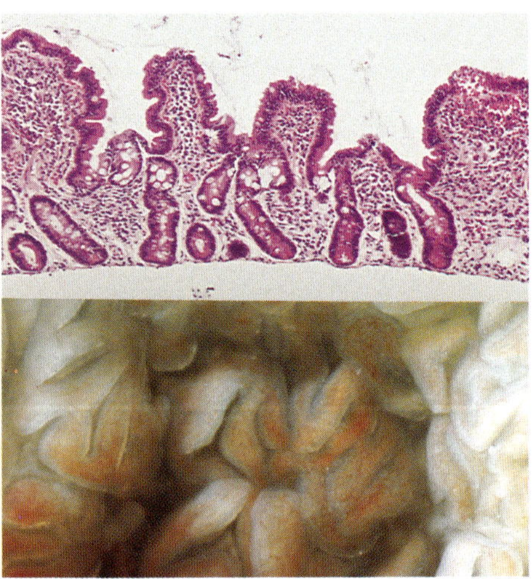

Fig. 2.67 Partial villous atrophy in tropical sprue. Top: Jejunal biopsy showing moderate partial villous atrophy. The villi are squat and the ratio of villus height to crypt depth approaches unity. ×70. H&E stain. Bottom: The dissecting microscope view shows the pattern of convolutions or ridges representing severe partial villous atrophy.

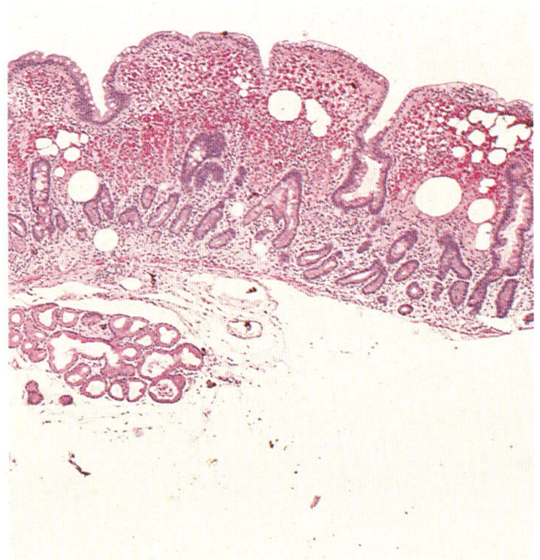

Fig. 2.68 Whipple's disease. Small intestinal biopsy. Subtotal villous atrophy with marked blunting of villi. By courtesy of Dr J. Cunningham

and intestinal biopsy, to exclude gluten enteropathy, Whipple's disease and lymphoma. Histopathological findings include broadening and shortening of the villi, with infiltration of the mucosa by chronic inflammatory cells (Fig. 2.67).

Treatment with folate alone often relieves the symptoms but usually does not restore intestinal morphology and function to normal. Addition of tetracycline and a vitamin B_{12} regimen usually results in prompt clinical improvement and eventual healing of the inflammatory lesion.

WHIPPLE'S DISEASE

Whipple's disease is a chronic multisystem disease in which the small intestine and associated lymph nodes are prominently involved. Diarrhoea is present in nearly all cases. Microscopic examination of the small intestine shows villous atrophy (Fig. 2.68), dilated lacteals containing fat droplets (Fig. 2.69), and large numbers of macrophages with foamy cytoplasm which contains many periodic acid–Schiff (PAS) positive 'sickle-form' particles (Figs. 2.70 & 2.71). Similar findings may be present

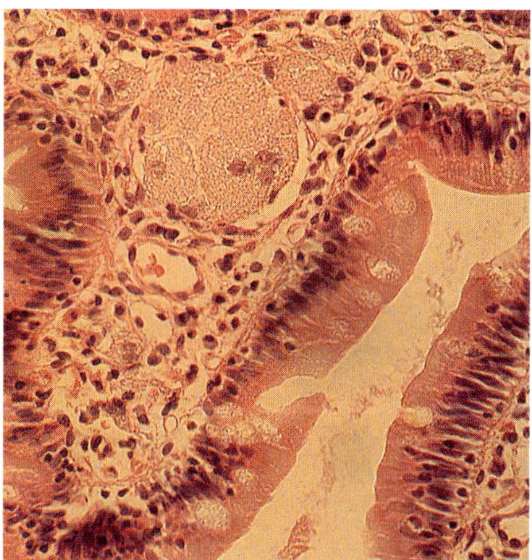

Fig. 2.69 Whipple's disease. Focus of large lipid-containing macrophages in the lamina propria of the intestine. PAS stain. By courtesy of Dr C. Edwards.

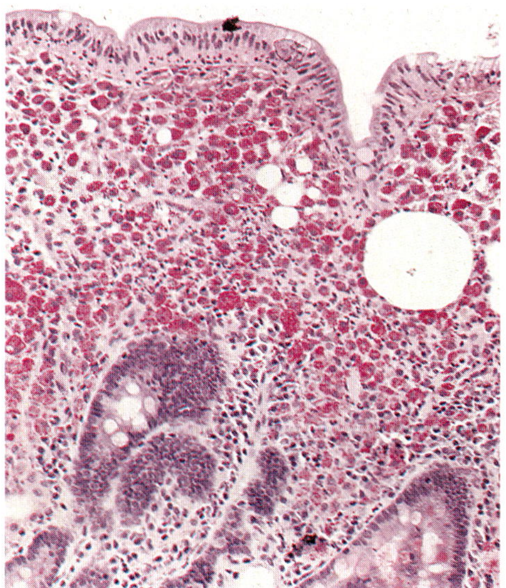

Fig. 2.70 Whipple's disease. High power view showing the diagnostic diastase-resistant PAS-positive material in submucosal macrophages. By courtesy of Dr J. Cunningham.

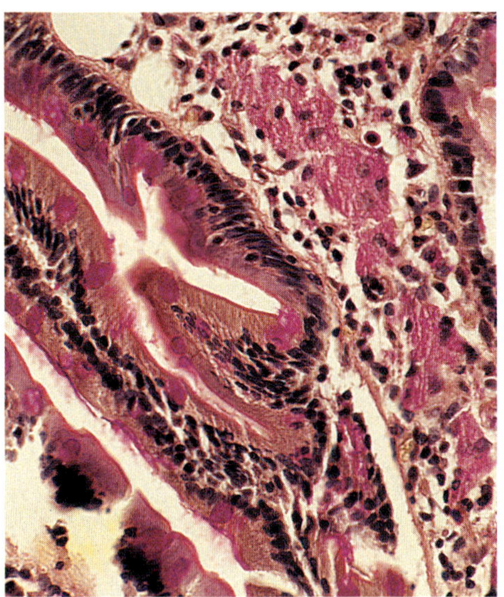

Fig. 2.71 Whipple's disease. Intestinal mucosa stained by the PAS reagent method showing typical PAS-positive material within large macrophages in the lamina propria. By courtesy of Dr C. Edwards.

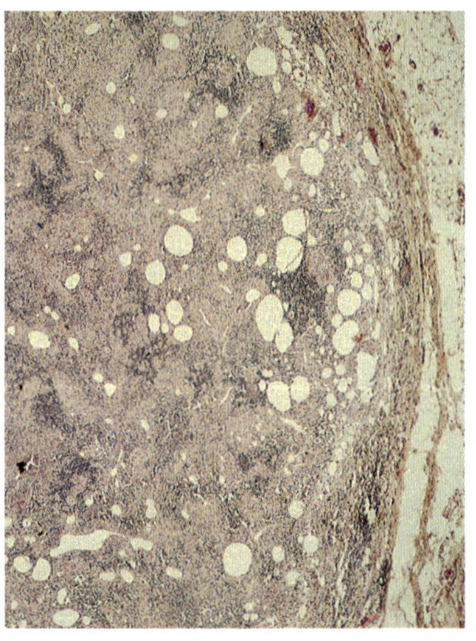 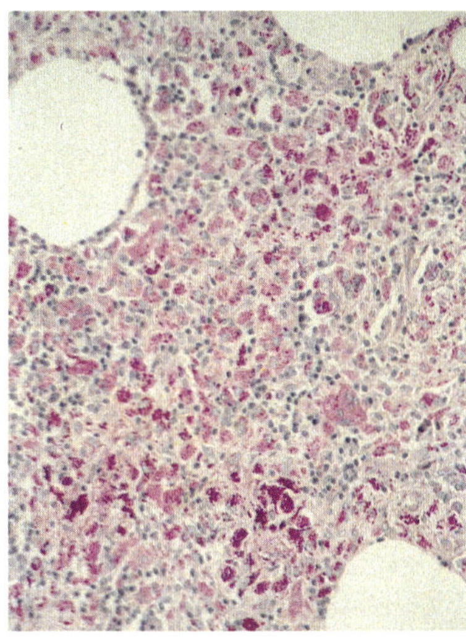

Fig. 2.72 Histological appearance of a lymph node with similar features to those in the small bowel. The architecture is distorted by the macrophage infiltrate and large vacuoles. Left: ×30. H&E stain. Right: ×180. PAS stain.

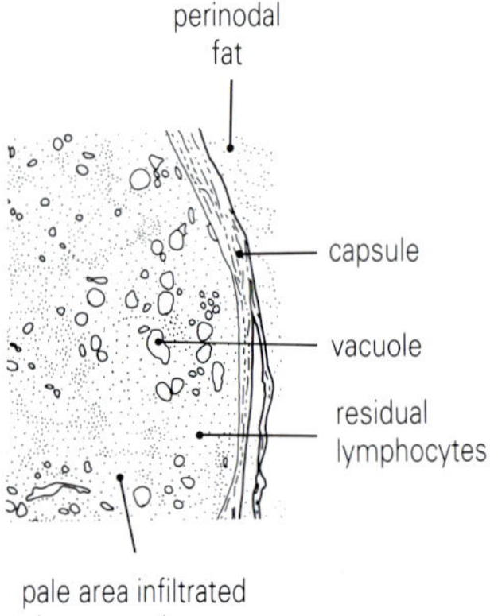

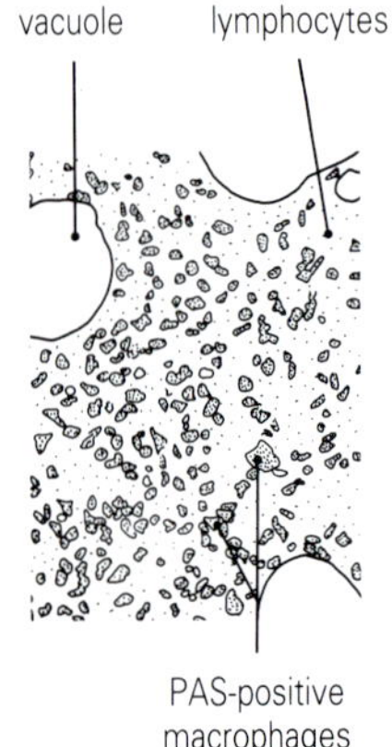

in the draining lymph nodes (Fig. 2.72). Electron microscopy reveals the presence in many tissues of small rod-shaped microorganisms, approximately 0.2 × 2.0 mm in size, with a homogenous cell wall (Fig. 2.73). These organisms are most abundant in the extracellular spaces of the lamina propria of the small intestine, but have been found in many other tissues of the body. Thus far it has not been possible to grow these organisms in culture or to transmit them to experimental animals. In addition to diarrhoea, a wide variety of other manifestations including fever, weight loss, anaemia, intermittent arthralgias, malabsorption, abdominal pain, lymphadenopathy, skin pigmentation, polyserositis, nonbacterial endocarditis, dementia and various neurological abnormalities may be present. Barium enema may reveal dilated jejunal loops with thickened, nodular folds (Fig. 2.74).

Many patients with Whipple's disease experience prompt remission of symptoms after treatment with antibiotics. In these patients the bacilli disappear from jejunal biopsy specimens and there is improvement in mucosal anatomy. A recommended regimen is penicillin plus streptomycin for two weeks, followed by oral tetracycline administration for approximately one year. About one-third of patients eventually relapse, but the average remission lasts for about 4 years. Treatment with tetracycline alone is less effective. Shorter courses of therapy are usually followed by early relapse. Many relapses after antimicrobial therapy involve the nervous system. This finding has led to the recommendation that patients receive an antibiotic that can cross the blood–brain barrier in the absence of meningeal inflammation, such as trimethoprim–sulphamethoxazole.

The underlying defect which allows the development of Whipple's disease is unknown. A good possibility is that the monocytes and macrophages of these individuals, although able to engulf the bacilli seen in this disease, are unable to destroy and digest them.

As noted above, involvement of the gut by MAI in patients with AIDS may mimic the clinical, histopathological and radiological findings of Whipple's disease.

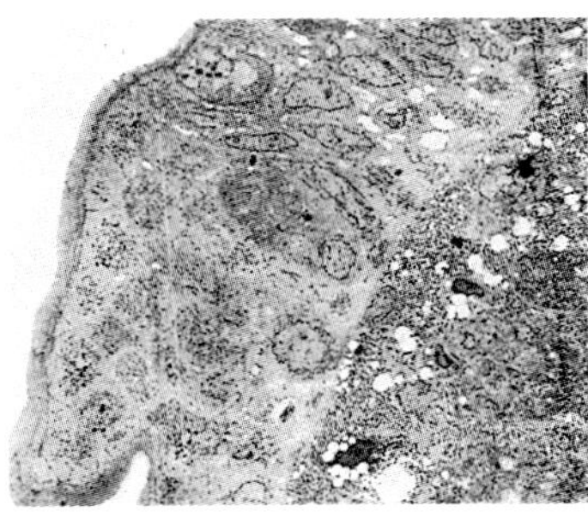

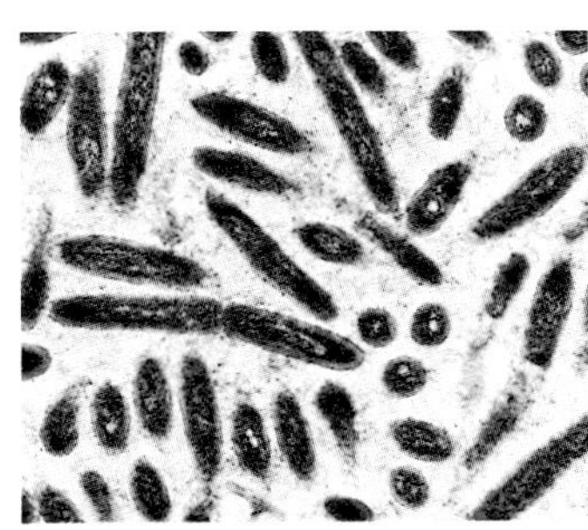

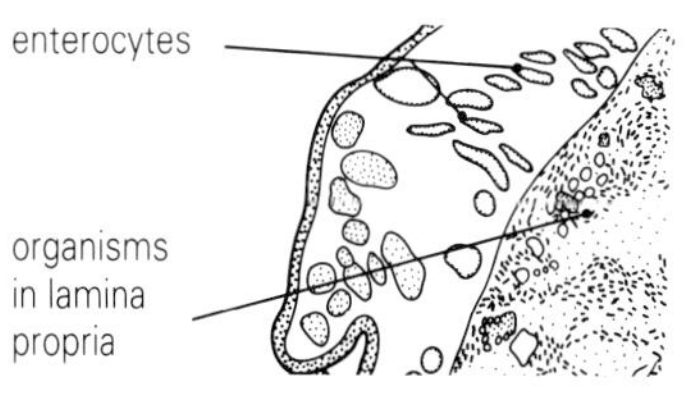

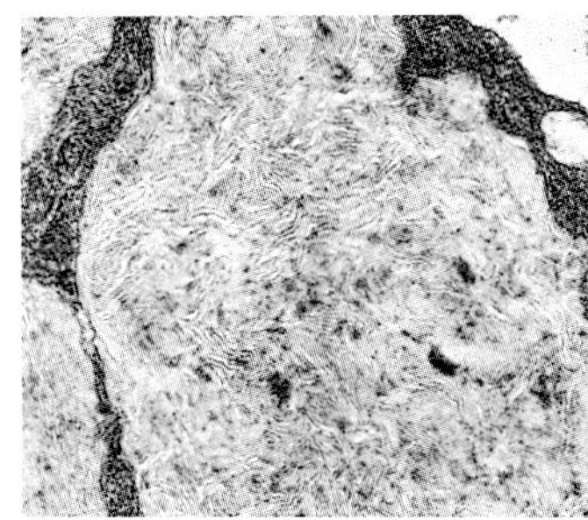

Fig. 2.73 Electron micrographs of Whipple's disease in the small intestine. Top left: Large numbers of rod-shaped organisms lying free in the lamina propria. ×700. Top right: Individual organisms under high power. ×14 000. Bottom right: Macrophage containing the empty shells of bacteria. Such cells persist long after the active disease state. ×14 000.

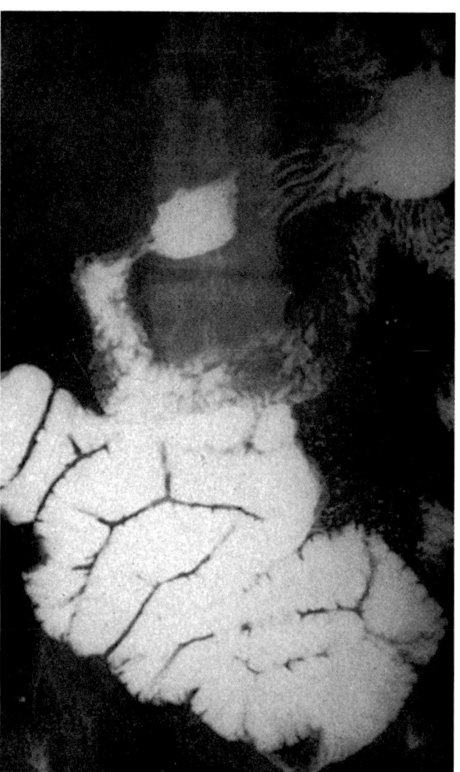

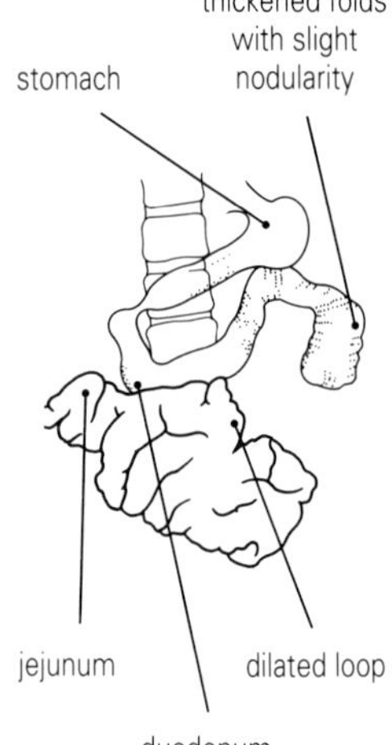

Fig. 2.74 Barium examination of the small intestine in Whipple's disease showing dilated jejunal loops with some thickened, slightly nodular folds proximally.

Chapter 3

Protozoal, Helminthic and Viral Enteric Infections

PROTOZOAL INFECTIONS

ENTAMOEBA HISTOLYTICA (AMOEBIASIS)

Entamoeba histolytica is a protozoan parasite which inhabits the wall and lumen of the human colon. It moves by means of pseudopodia and feeds by phagocytosis. There is still debate about whether or not a non-invasive form, which inhabits only the lumen of the gut and is incapable of damaging the tissues, also exists. The life cycle of this organism is relatively simple. The motile trophozoites invade the bowel wall and also inhabit the lumen. Under certain conditions the trophozoite undergoes encystment within the lumen of the bowel. The cyst passes out of the host in the faeces and, if ingested, passes through the stomach unharmed to reach the small intestine. There it undergoes cell division and conversion into a trophozoite. The cyst form is responsible for transmission via contaminated water or vegetables or by direct faecal–oral spread.

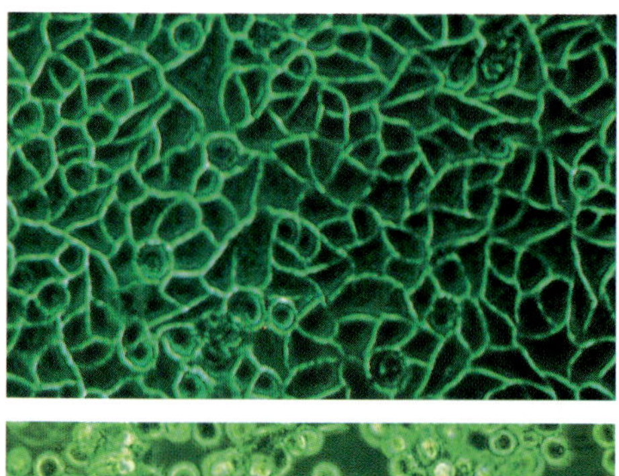

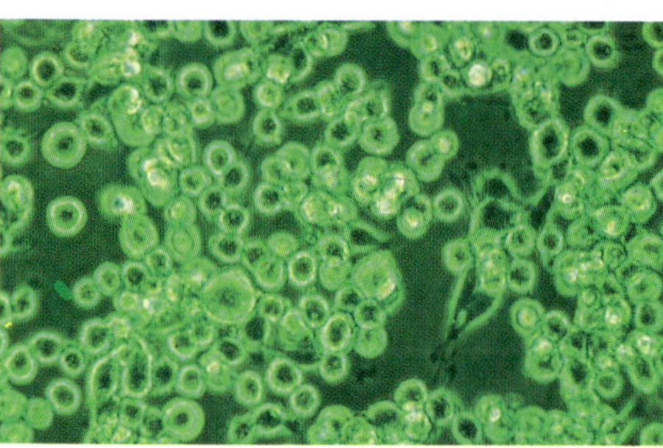

Fig. 3.1 Amoebic colitis. HeLa cell assay for *Entamoeba histolytica* cytotoxin showing normal cell monolayer (top) and cells after exposure to the toxin (bottom). Note the disruption of the monolayer and the rounding up of cells. By courtesy of Dr F. Pittman.

Fig. 3.2 Amoebic colitis. Colon showing discrete ulcerations with surrounding oedema and hyperaemia. (Compare with shigellosis where the entire mucosa is inflamed.) By courtesy of Prof. M. S. R. Hutt.

Approximately 10% of the world's population is infected with *E. histolytica*, and more than 10 million cases of invasive amoebiasis occur each year. The prevalence depends upon factors which determine the opportunities for transmission; these factors include sanitation, degree of crowding, socioeconomic status and cultural habits. In some countries 40–50% of individuals may be infected. In the USA the overall prevalence of infection is approximately 4%; however, it is as high as 70% in institutions for the mentally retarded and is about 30% among male homosexuals in New York City.

Incidence is also high among migrant workers, immigrants and travellers from endemic areas.

E. histolytica adheres to intestinal mucosal cells by means of specific receptors and produces cytotoxic factors (Fig. 3.1) which enable it to invade the colon with lysis of the mucosal cells. The lesions in the colon range from a non-specific colitis to flask-shaped ulcers which may extend through the mucosa and muscularis mucosae into the submucosa (Figs 3.2 & 3.3). Microscopic examination reveals trophozoites of *E. histolytica* and inflammatory cells in the lamina propria (Figs 3.4, 3.5 & 3.6)

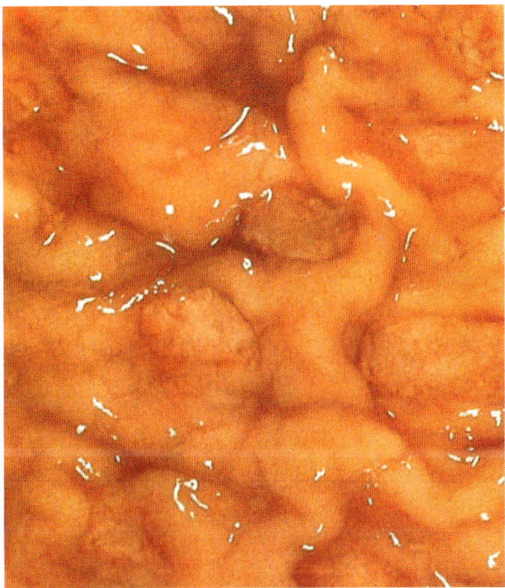

Fig. 3.3 Macroscopic appearance of the colonic surface showing amoebic ulcers. By courtesy of Dr S. Lucas.

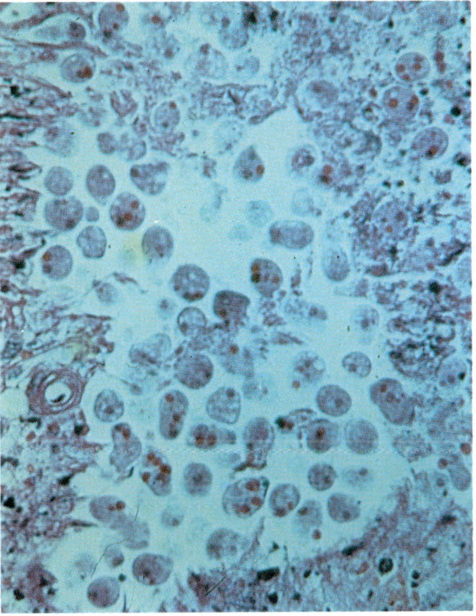

Fig. 3.4 Amoebic colitis. Histological section of bowel wall showing trophozoites of *Entamoeba histolytica*, many containing ingested red blood cells. Due to the shrinkage artifact, the amoebae appear to be lying within a space. H&E stain. By courtesy of Dr K. Juniper.

and on the epithelial surface (Figs 3.7 & 3.8). In the tissue the rounded amoebae are surrounded by a halo which is a result of fixation artifact; the organisms may be distinguished from the host cells by the nuclear morphology, PAS staining and the presence of intracellular erythrocytes (Fig. 3.9). Cell-mediated immunity appears to be more important than humoral immunity in prevention of recurrence of invasive colonic or hepatic disease.

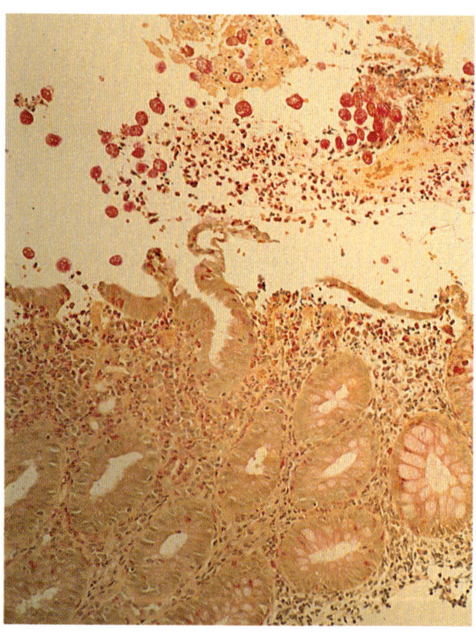

Fig. 3.5 Amoebic colitis. Section of colon showing trophozoites of *Entamoeba histolytica* (stained magenta with the PAS reagent method) embedded in purulent material in the lumen, and an inflammatory infiltrate composed primarily of polymorphonuclear leucocytes in the lamina propria. The lysosomes of the PMN leucocytes also stain magenta with the PAS reagent method. By courtesy of Dr C. Edwards.

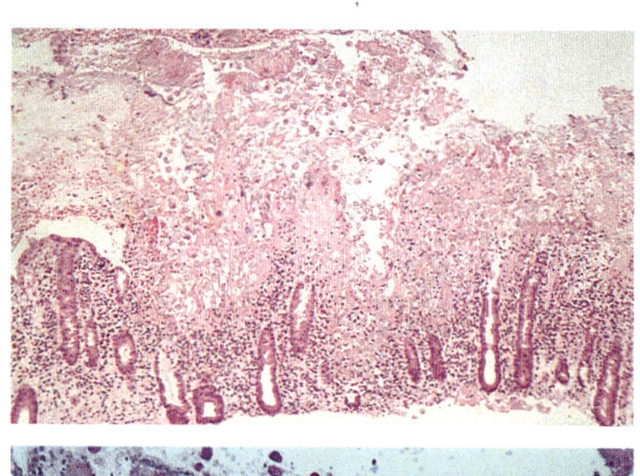

Fig. 3.6 Rectal biopsy in amoebiasis. Top: Invasion of the mucosa can be seen as well as many organisms in the surface debris. ×75. H&E stain. Bottom: Surface debris should be examined carefully, as it may be the only site at which organisms are found. Periodic acid–Schiff reagent stains amoebae magenta; it is the best way of detecting small numbers of organisms. ×180. PAS stain.

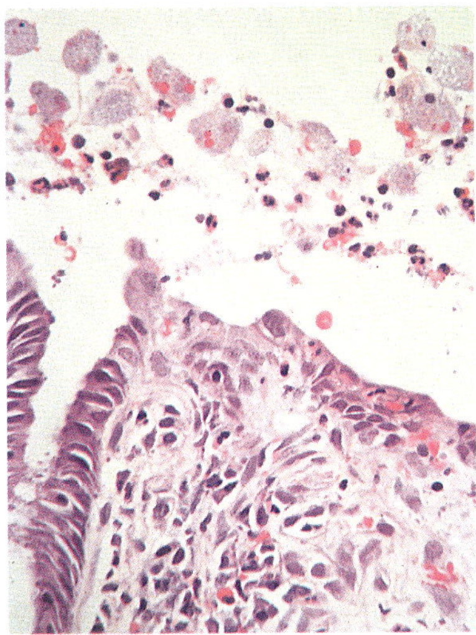

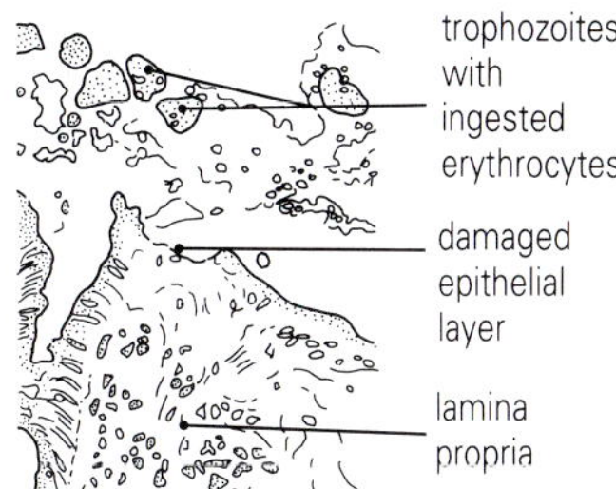

Fig. 3.7 Amoebic colitis. Intestinal biopsy showing loss of mucosal lining cells and sparse infiltrate of inflammatory cells in the lamina propria. Trophozoites and polymorphs are present in the lumen. H&E stain.

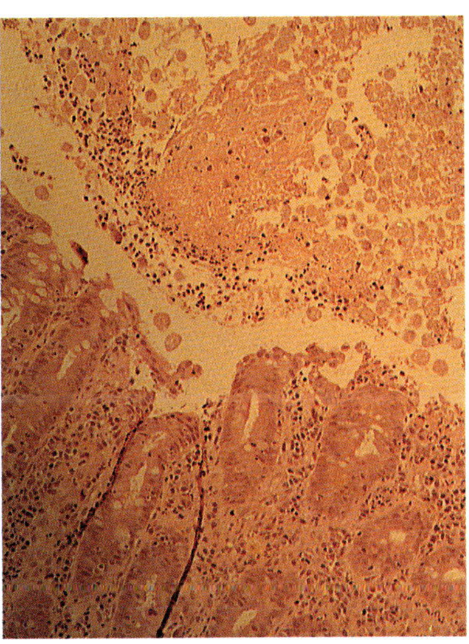

Fig. 3.8 Amoebic colitis. Biopsy of colon showing numerous organisms embedded in fibrin and necrotic material in the lumen, with an acute inflammatory infiltrate composed predominantly of polymorphonuclear leucocytes. By courtesy of Dr C. Edwards.

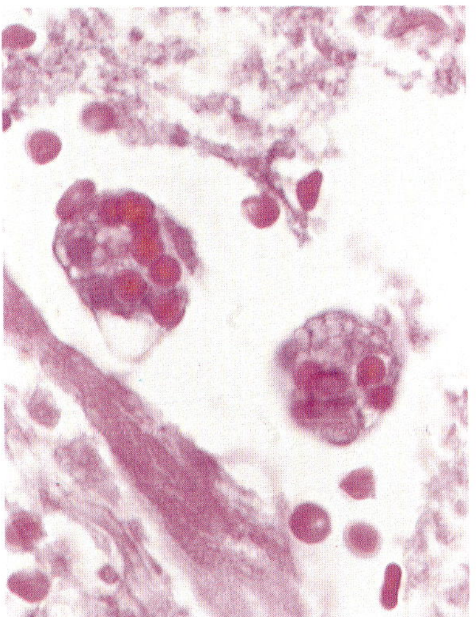

Fig. 3.9 Amoebae with ingested erythrocytes. ×660. H&E stain. By courtesy of Dr S. Lucas.

Asymptomatic infection is the most common form of infection with *E. histolytica*. The spectrum of illness produced by this organism is very broad. The most common type is chronic, mild, intermittent diarrhoea with colicky abdominal pain. More severe diarrhoeal disease may also occur with fever, dysentery (blood, mucus and pus in the stool – Fig. 3.10) and severe abdominal pain and tenderness.

Massive infection may be complicated by development of an acute surgical abdomen with severe abdominal pain and distension, vomiting and absent bowel sounds due to perforation of the bowel and combined amoebic and bacterial peritonitis. Toxic megacolon occurs occasionally, especially in patients who have been receiving corticosteroid therapy. Amoeboma, usually occurring in

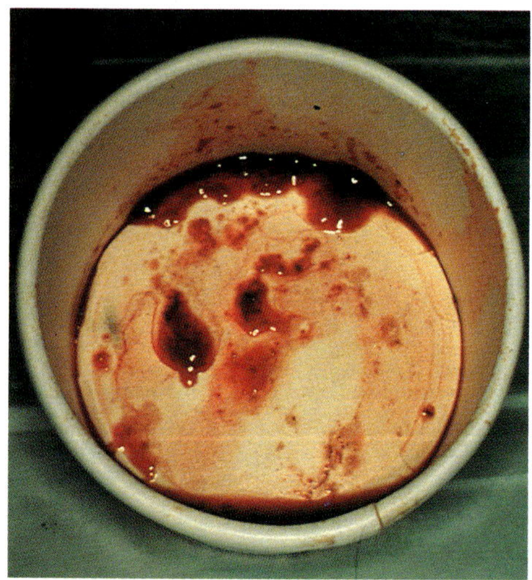

Fig. 3.10 Amoebic colitis. Typical dysentery stool (small volume, blood and mucus) from a patient with acute amoebiasis. By courtesy of Dr H. L. DuPont.

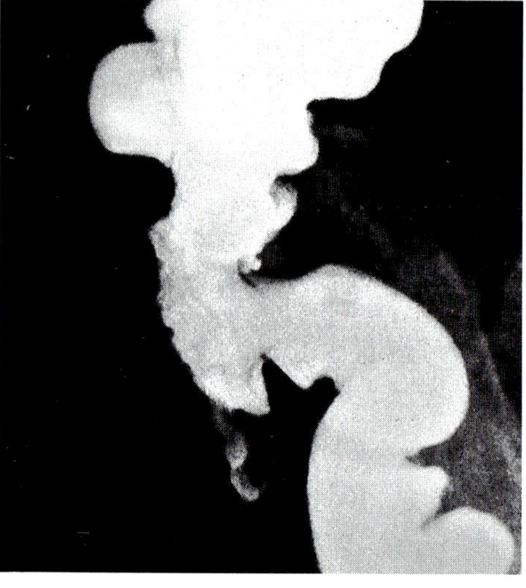

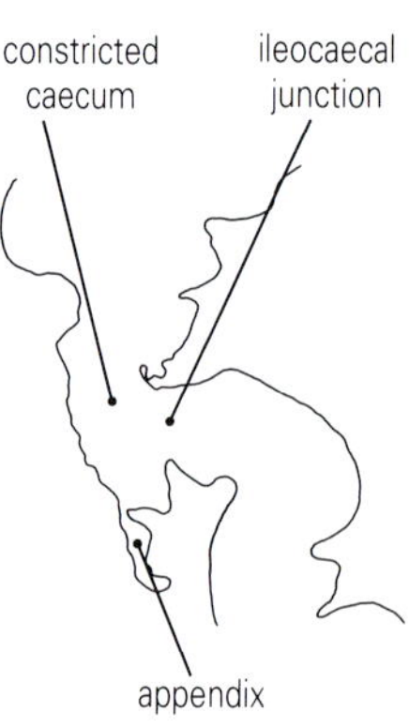

Fig. 3.11 Amoebic colitis. Barium study showing amoeboma of caecum. Note constriction and distortion of the caecal region. By courtesy of Dr F. Pittman.

the caecum and ascending colon, may manifest as an annular lesion mimicking carcinoma of the colon or as a palpable mass which resembles a pyogenic abscess (Figs 3.11, 3.12 & 3.13). Chronic intermittent diarrhoea lasting for more than a year may follow an episode of acute amoebic colitis and may resemble non-infectious inflammatory bowel disease.

Extraintestinal infection most often involves the liver (see Chapter 5). From the liver, infection may extend into the pleural space with production of empyema and lung abscess, or into the pericardium. Rarely, brain abscess may occur. In extraintestinal infection there may be no evidence of active amoebic colitis, and the stools may be negative for amoebae.

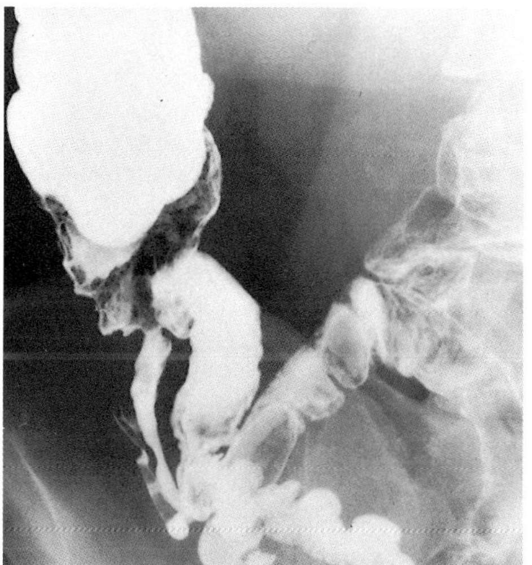

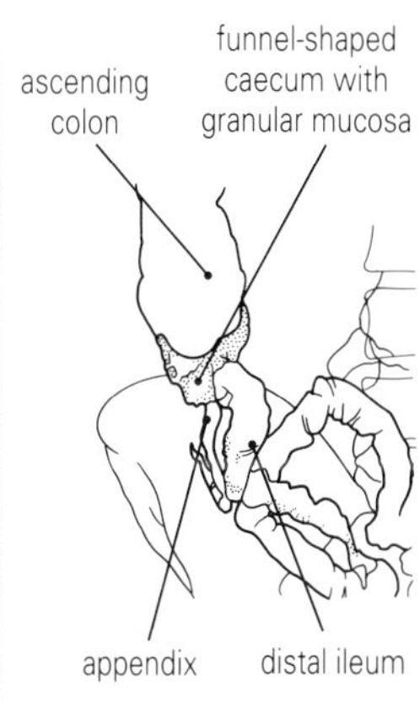

Fig. 3.12 Barium enema radiograph in chronic amoebic colitis showing a funnel-shaped caecum with granular deformity.

Fig. 3.13 Barium enema showing an amoeboma in the ascending colon.

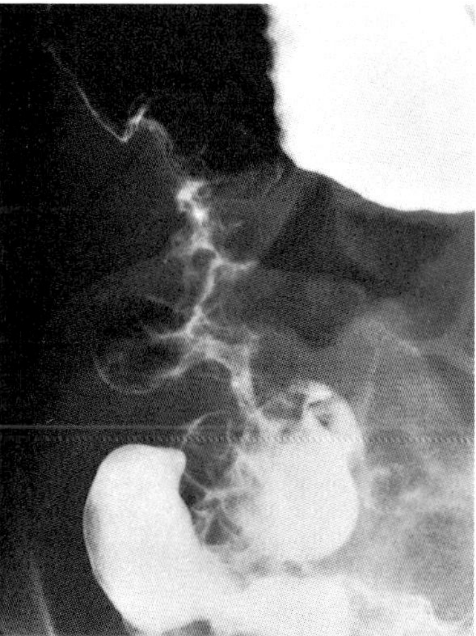

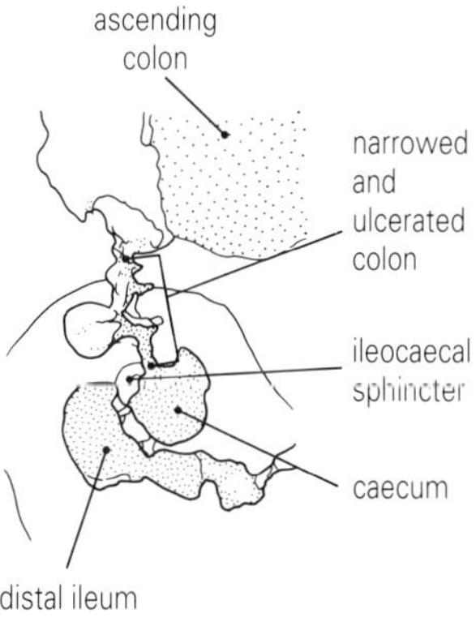

In intestinal infection, the diagnosis is made by identifying either cysts (Fig. 3.14) or trophozoites (Fig. 3.15) of *E. histolytica* in the stool. Fresh material from a lesion seen at sigmoidoscopy may be suspended in saline and examined on a warm microscope stage for trophozoites. Trophozoites may also be identified in smears stained with iron–haematoxylin or Wheatley's trichrome stains. A stool specimen may be suspended in a formalin–ether solution and the cysts concentrated at the formalin–ether interface by centrifugation and identified after staining with diluted iodine solution. A few laboratories are able to culture *E. histolytica* from clinical specimens. At least three stool specimens should be examined; administration of a saline purge can increase the yield of positive examinations.

Sigmoidoscopy usually reveals a hyperaemic, oedematous mucosa with punctate haemorrhages and small ulcers (Fig. 3.16). The large confluent ulcers described in textbooks are seen less often (Figs 3.17 & 3.18). In early infections the mucosa may appear normal.

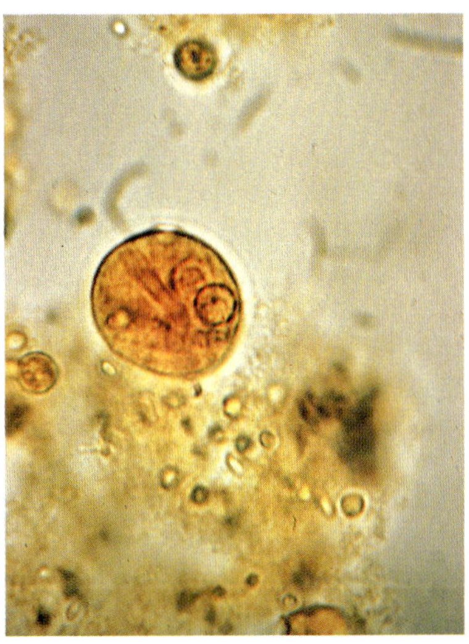

Fig. 3.14 Amoebic colitis. Cyst of *Entamoeba histolytica* showing round shape, refractile wall and multiple nuclei. Iodine stain.

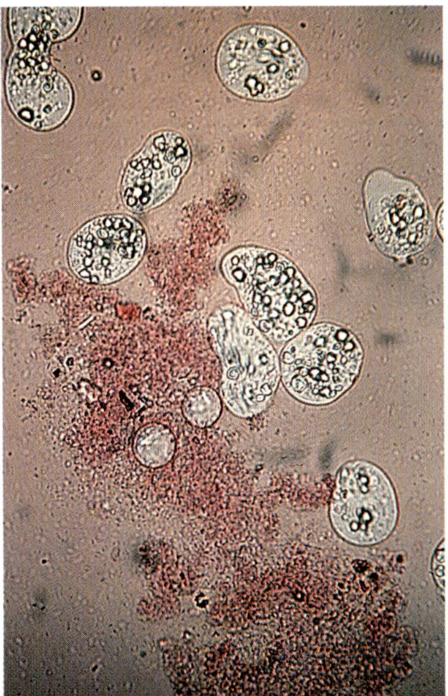

Fig. 3.15 Amoebic colitis. Trophozoites of *Entamoeba histolytica* showing amoeboid form and internal organelles. Eosin stain.

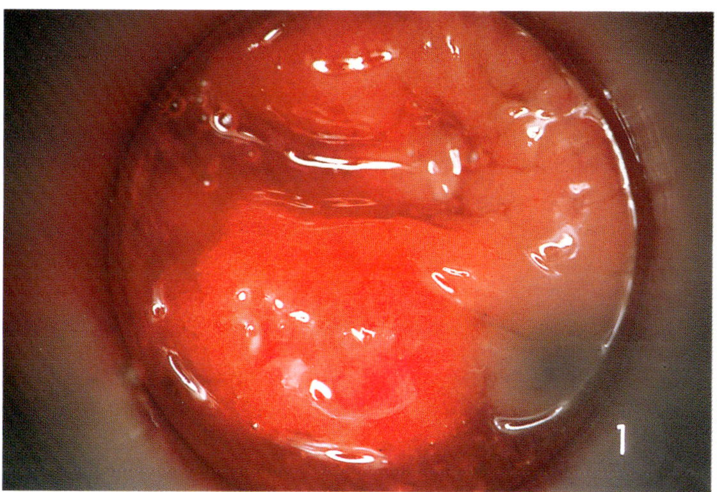

Fig. 3.16 Amoebic colitis. Sigmoidoscopic view of colonic mucosa in a typical case of amoebic dysentery showing the non-ulcerated diffuse colitis which is the predominant form of the disease. By courtesy of Dr R. H. Gilman.

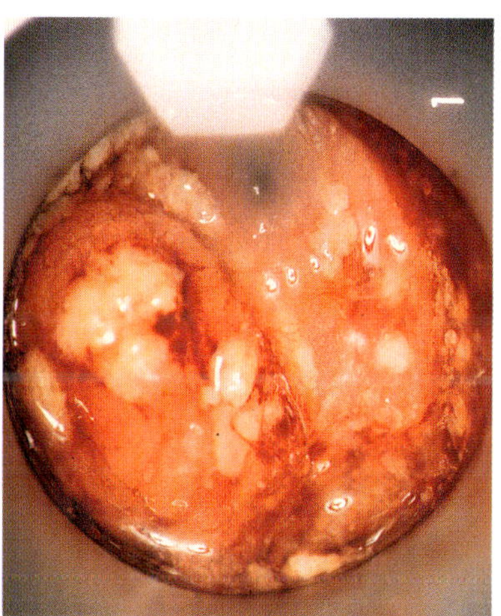

Fig. 3.17 Amoebic colitis. Sigmoidoscopic view of colonic mucosa showing the 'textbook', but less common form of amoebic dysentery, with deep ulcers and over-lying purulent exudate. By courtesy of Dr R.H. Gilman.

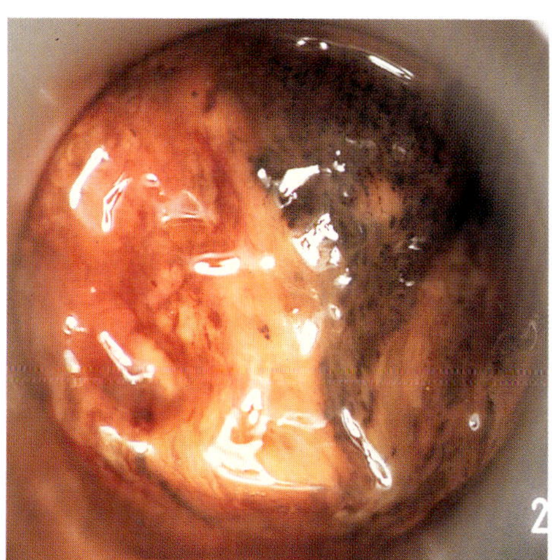

Fig. 3.18 Amoebic colitis. Sigmoidoscopic view of colonic mucosa showing extensive ulceration with a 'Dyak hair ulcer'. By courtesy of Dr R.H. Gilman.

The indirect fluorescent antibody test is usually negative in asymptomatic cyst passers, but is positive in approximately 85% of cases of invasive amoebic colitis and is nearly always positive in amoebic liver abscess.

The optimum treatment regimen varies with the type of disease being treated. Asymptomatic intraluminal infection can be treated with tetracycline in combination with either diiodohydroxyquin or diloxanide furoate. Invasive intestinal disease should be treated with metronidazole followed by treatment with either diiodohydroxyquin or diloxanide furoate. Extraintestinal infection may be treated with the same regimens used in the treatment of invasive intestinal disease. Since a few liver abscesses are not cured with metronidazole plus diiodohydroxyquin or diloxanide furoate, some authorities would add treatment with chloroquine.

GIARDIASIS

Giardia lamblia is a flagellated protozoan which is a major cause of diarrhoeal disease throughout the world. The organism exists as a free-living trophozoite and as a thin-walled cyst form. Infection is acquired by ingesting the cysts, usually in faecally contaminated water. The disease is a common cause of chronic debilitating diarrhoea in travellers. Well-publicized outbreaks have occurred in visitors to St. Petersburg and among campers and hikers in western states of the USA. *G. lamblia* infects many animal species including beavers, which may contaminate the water of mountain streams. Up to 50% of children in day-care centres may be infected and the organism is readily spread to family members. Infection is also common among homosexual men and in crowded custodial institutions.

The organism adheres by means of its disc to the brush border of the small intestine (Figs 3.19 & 3.20), sometimes disrupting the integrity of the brush border. *G. lamblia* apparently does not produce an enterotoxin and the mechanism by which it causes diarrhoea is not fully understood. Both cell-mediated and humoral mechanisms appear to be important in recovery from disease and in resistance to infection with *G. lamblia*. Patients with common variable immunodeficiency and X-linked agammaglobulinaemia are predisposed to infection with this organism, and selective IgA deficiency may also increase susceptibility to infection.

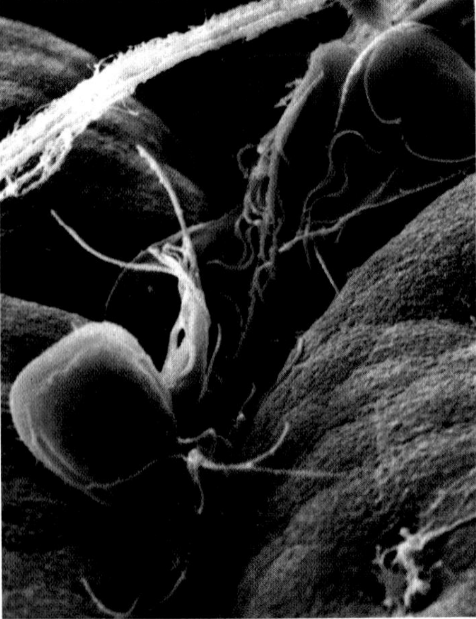

Fig. 3.19 Giardiasis. Scanning electron micrograph of *Giardia lamblia* trophozoites in a crevice of a human jejunal villus. The slightly concave ventral adhesive disc and ventral flagella are seen in the organism upper right; the irregular dorsal surface can be seen in the giardia lower left. ×1550. By courtesy of Dr R.L. Owen.

Infection with *G. lamblia* may result in asymptomatic cyst passage, an acute self-limited episode of diarrhoea, or chronic diarrhoea with malabsorption and weight loss (Fig. 3.21). Symptomatic patients usually have diarrhoea, with stools that are greasy, foul smelling and may float, as well as abdominal cramps, bloating and flatulence, anorexia, malaise and nausea.

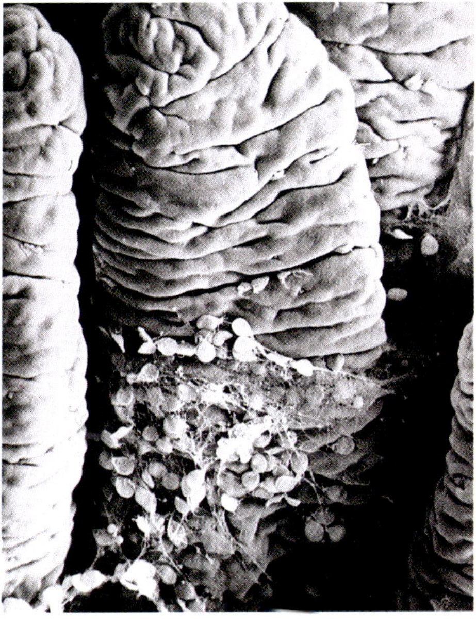

Fig. 3.20 Electron micrograph showing villi of the mouse jejunum with *Giardia lamblia* trophozoites adhering to the surface near the bases of the villi, wedged into furrows and lying in mucus. By courtesy of Dr R. L. Owen.

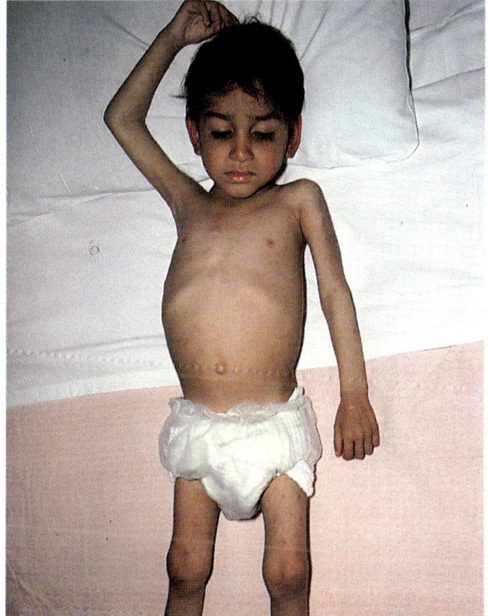

Fig. 3.21 Giardiasis. Child with chronic severe infection with *Giardia lamblia,* showing abdominal distension and evidence of malnutrition.

Diagnosis is made by finding the organism in the stools or in duodenal aspirate or biopsy material. Liquid stool may be examined directly in a wet mount for the motile trophozoites or cysts (Fig. 3.22). Fresh stool or stool preserved in polyvinyl alcohol may be stained with iron–haematoxylin or trichrome stains. Organisms are found in only about 50% of cases when a single stool specimen is examined. If three stools are examined the detection rate approaches 90%. If stools are negative,

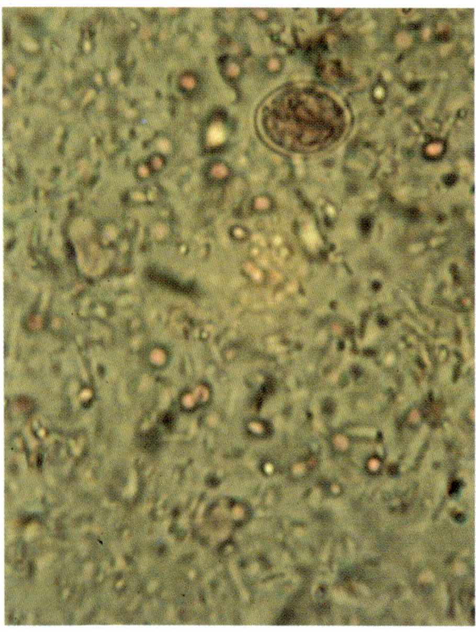

Fig. 3.22 Giardiasis. Cyst of *Giardia lamblia* showing ovoid shape, prominent cyst wall, granular cytoplasm and at least two nuclei. By courtesy of Dr H. L. DuPont.

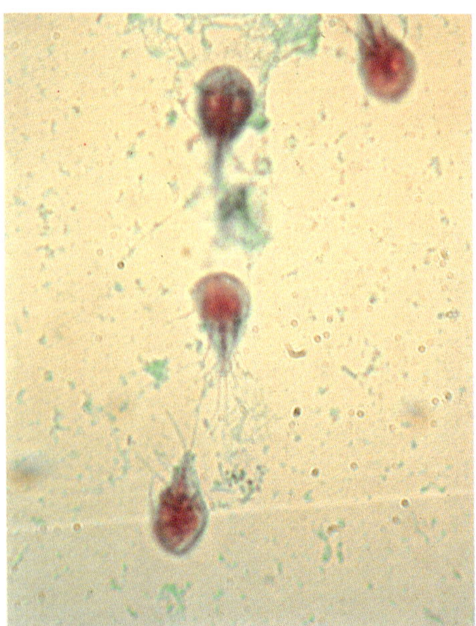

Fig. 3.23 Giardiasis. Trophozoites of *Giardia lamblia* obtained from mucus stripped from an Enterotest string pulled from the duodenum after overnight passage. Note the characteristic shape, paired nuclei and multiple flagella. The patient also had adult acquired hypogammaglobulinaemia. Three stool examinations for *Giardia* had been negative. Trichrome stain. By courtesy of Dr F. Pittman.

duodenal material may be sampled by the Enterotest technique. In this test a nylon string is contained in a gelatin capsule; the free end of the string is secured at the mouth and the capsule is swallowed. After 4–6 hours, or overnight, the string is removed and examined fresh under a wet mount or stained (Fig. 3.23). Examination of aspirated duodenal fluid, duodenal brushings or biopsy specimens may also provide the diagnosis.

Both quinacrine and metronidazole are highly effective in the treatment of giardiasis. Provision of a safe water supply and maintenance of good personal hygiene will prevent transmission of this infection. Travellers in endemic areas should boil water for one minute before drinking, or add halazone (5 tablets per litre) and allow to stand for 30 minutes before drinking.

CRYPTOSPORIDIOSIS

Until recently, *Cryptosporidium* species were thought to be an uncommon cause of mild diarrhoeal disease, occurring primarily in children. Improved techniques for detecting the organism in stool specimens have shown that this infection is relatively common and, in some localities, that it is the most common enteric protozoan infection. In immunocompetent individuals this organism usually causes asymptomatic infection or a transient watery diarrhoea lasting up to ten days, accompanied by abdominal cramps and nausea. Both the symptoms and faecal excretion of organisms subside without antimicrobial treatment. More recently, infection by *Cryptosporidium* species has been found to be a major opportunistic infection in patients with AIDS. Infection in these patients usually results in a relentless, progressive, watery diarrhoea which persists until death. Occasional patients have appeared to respond to therapy, especially with spiramycin, but no treatment has been consistently effective. Involvement of the biliary tract sometimes occurs in patients with AIDS, resulting in a picture of acute biliary colic.

Diagnosis of cryptosporidiosis is made by finding the oocysts in the faeces, using either modified acid fast stains (Fig. 3.24) or iodine stains. The cryptosporidia are acid-fast, but iodine negative. These minute organisms (2–4 mm) may also sometimes be seen lining intestinal epithelial cells in small bowel biopsy specimens (Figs 3.25, 3.26 & 3.27).

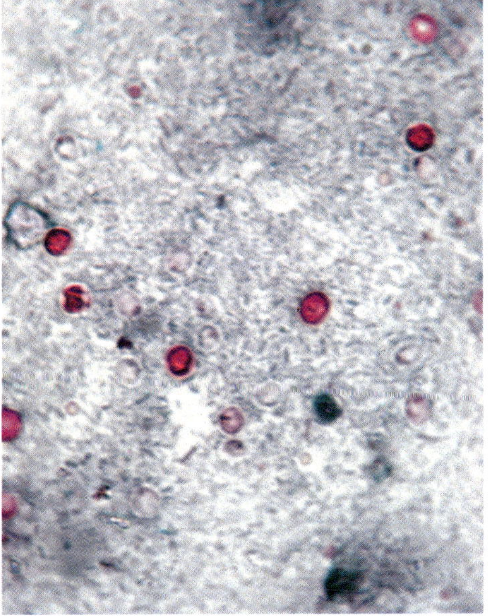

Fig. 3.24 Cryptosporidiosis. Modified acid-fast stain of stool specimen showing characteristic acid-fast *Cryptosporidium* organisms.

ISOSPORA BELLI

Like organisms of the genus *Cryptosporidium*, *Isospora belli* is a coccidian protozoan parasite which usually produces a mild self-limited diarrhoeal disease in immunocompetent patients, but can produce a severe progressive disease in patients with AIDS (Fig. 3.28). The infection is diagnosed by finding the large (20–30 mm) ellipsoidal acid-fast oocysts in the faeces (Fig. 3.29). However, *Isospora belli* infection is not a zoonosis. It usually responds promptly to treatment with either oral trimethoprim–sulphamethoxazole or pyrimethamine–sulphadoxine.

MICROSPORIDIOSIS

Microsporidia are small (4×5 mm), primitive, intracellular spore-forming protozoa which lack mitochondria. Recently one species, *Enterocytozoon bieneusi*, has been implicated as a cause of chronic diarrhoea and weight loss in patients with HIV

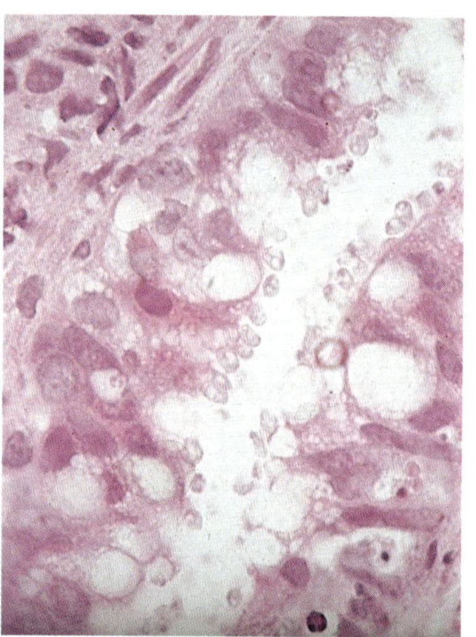

Fig. 3.25 Cryptosporidiosis. Numerous organisms in the brush border of the intestine. By courtesy of Dr J. Newman.

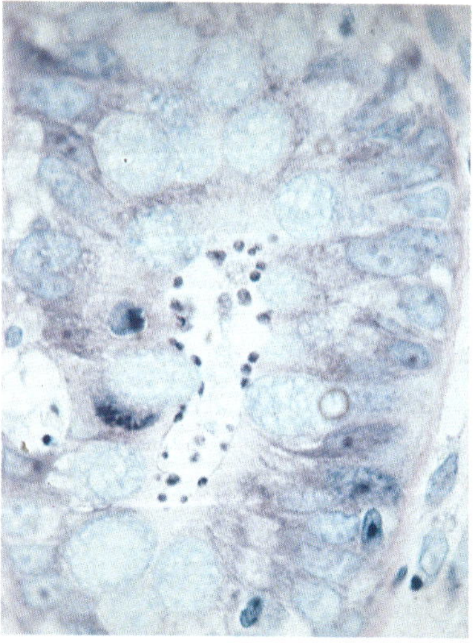

Fig. 3.26 Cryptosporidiosis, with numerous organisms in the brush border of the intestine. Giemsa stain. By courtesy of Dr J. Newman.

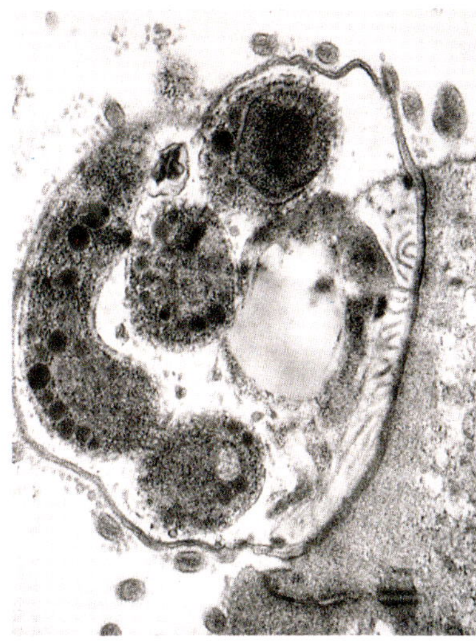

Fig. 3.27 Cryptosporidiosis. Electron micrograph showing mature schizont with several merozoites attached to the intestinal epithelium.

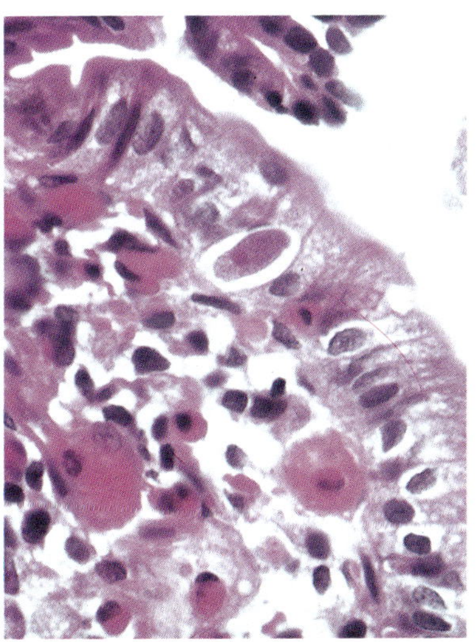

Fig. 3.28 Human coccidiosis. Enteric infection in a patient with AIDS. A single *Isospora belli* organism is seen within an epithelial cell, and there is a chronic inflammatory reaction in the lamina propria. By courtesy of Dr G. N. Griffin.

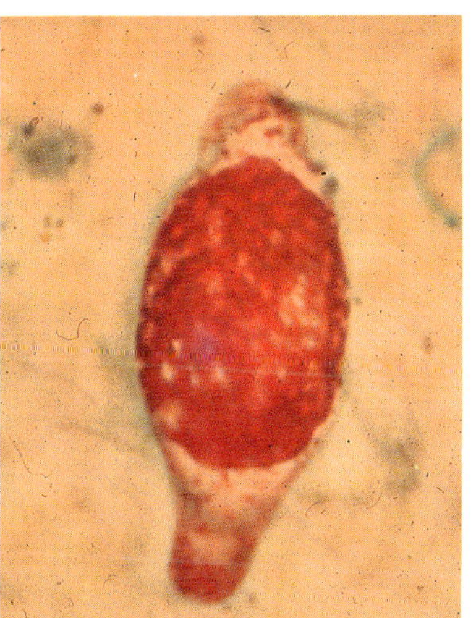

Fig. 3.29 *Isospora belli*. Oocyst in faeces. Modified acid-fast stain. By courtesy of Dr G. N. Griffin.

infection. The diagnosis can be made by finding the parasites or spores, by light or electron microscopy (Fig. 3.30), within enterocytes of the small bowel, or by detection of spores in faeces or duodenal aspirates stained with a modified trichrome stain. Preliminary studies indicate that this infection may be as frequent as cryptosporidiosis in patients with AIDS.

BALANTIDIUM COLI

Balantidium coli is a very large (100 mm) oval-

shaped ciliated protozoan that causes disease in a number of different mammalian species. Human disease usually occurs in individuals who have close contact with swine. The organism penetrates the mucosa of the colon and multiplies in the submucosa, producing a colitis with blood and mucus in the stool (dysentery). The diagnosis is made by finding the very large cysts or trophozoites in the stool or in biopsy specimens of the bowel (Figs 3.31 & 3.32). The infection can be treated with tetracycline, metronidazole or paromomycin.

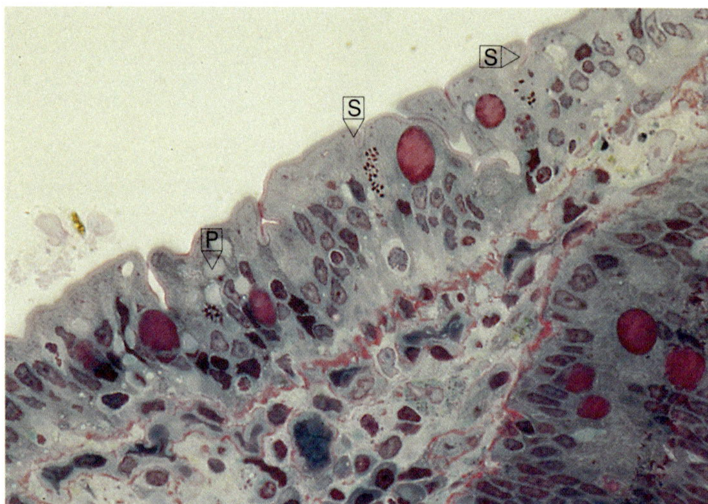

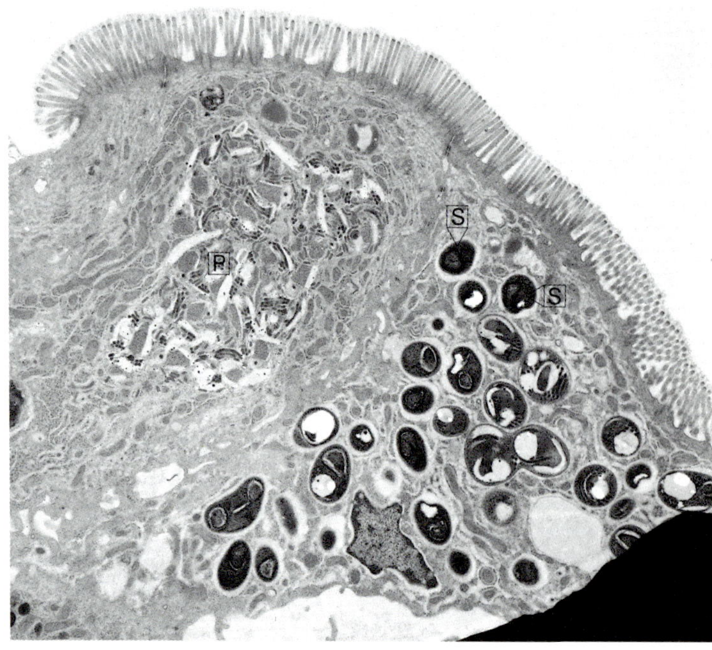

Fig. 3.30 Microsporidiosis. Upper: Duodenal biopsy showing lightly-stained oval parasites (P), clusters of densely-stained spores (S), and intraepithelial lymphocytes. ×320. Methylene blue-azure II, basic fuchsin stain. By courtesy of Dr J. M. Orenstein and W. B. Saunders Co. Lower: Transmission electron micrograph showing numerous sporoblasts (two not completed separation) and spores (S) present in the cytoplasm of an enterocyte. The adjacent cell contains a late sporogonial plasmodium (P) with numerous nuclei, developing polar tubes and electron-lucent clefts. ×4000. By courtesy of Dr J.M. Orenstein.

BLASTOCYSTIS HOMINIS

This organism, originally identified as a trichomonad, then long considered a yeast, has finally been identified as a sporozoan protozoan. It is commonly found in intestinal contents of healthy individuals. Its status as a human pathogen is controversial, and many patients who have diarrhoeal disease ascribed to *B. hominis* also have other, better-established enteric pathogens present concomitantly. However, recent reports have associated it with diarrhoea in severely immunocompromised patients, including several patients with AIDS. In a few cases the diarrhoea has responded to treatment with diiodohydroxyquin.

SCHISTOSOMIASIS

The schistosomes or blood flukes are parasitic flatworms. Three species are important causes of human infection: *Schistosoma mansoni*, *S. japonicum* and *S. haematobium*. Together they infect more than 200 million people worldwide and the incidence of human infection is increasing. The adult forms of *S. mansoni* and *S. japonicum* inhabit the portal and mesenteric veins; *S. haematobium* inhabits the vesical plexus of the bladder. Man is the principal definitive host for these three species of schistosomes. The worm lives in the venous system of the

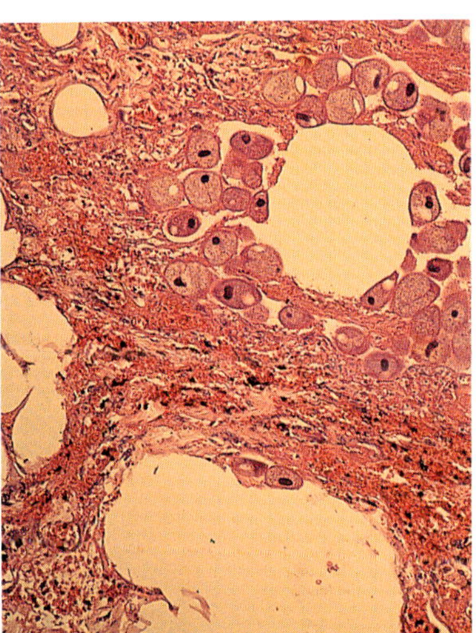

Fig. 3.31 Balantidiasis. Numerous large trophozoites in the wall of the intestine in a patient with AIDS.

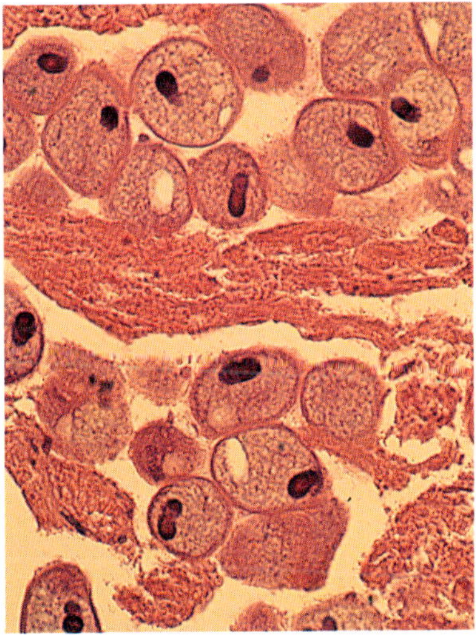

Fig. 3.32 Balantidiasis. Higher magnification showing typical foamy cytoplasm and bean-shaped macronucleus of *B. coli*. By courtesy of Dr J. Newman.

intestines (Fig. 3.33). The female worm inhabits a groove in the lateral edge of the body of the male (Fig. 3.34) and produces approximately 300 (*S. mansoni*) or 3000 (*S. japonicum*) eggs every day. These find their way into the lumen of the bowel and are excreted in the faeces (Fig. 3.35). In fresh water the eggs hatch and release motile ciliated miracidia which penetrate the body of the intermediate host, usually a snail of the genus *Biomphalaria* (*S. mansoni*) or *Oncomelania* (*S. japonicum*). The miracidia multiply asexually inside the snail; within a few weeks, hundreds of motile fork-tailed cercariae emerge. When the cercariae encounter human skin they penetrate it, lose their tails and change into schistosomula forms which migrate to the lungs and liver. In approximately 6 weeks they mature into adult worms which mate and pass through the venous system to their final habitat, where they may live for up to 10 years.

The geographical range of each species of schistosome is determined primarily by two factors: the presence of the specific snail that is the intermediate host; and the method of disposal of human excreta. *S. mansoni* occurs in Arabia, Africa, South America and many Caribbean islands. *S. japonicum* is found in China, Japan, and the Philippines. *S. haematobium* occurs in Africa and the Middle East.

Three major disease syndromes occur in schistosomiasis: schistosome dermatitis; katayama fever; and chronic schistosomiasis.

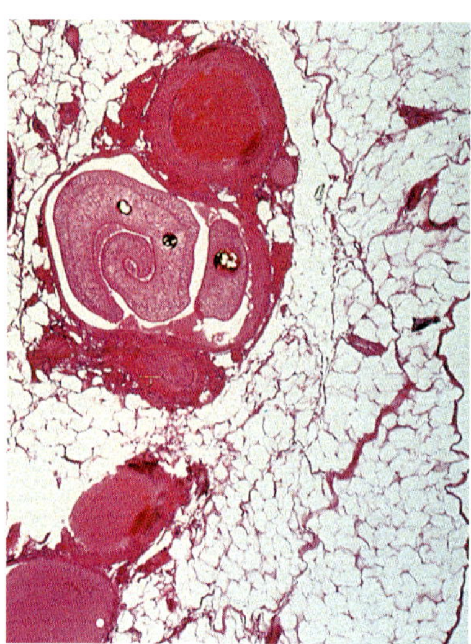

Fig. 3.33 Schistosomiasis. Section of mesentery showing adult *Schistosoma mansoni* worm lodged in the mesenteric vein. H&E stain.

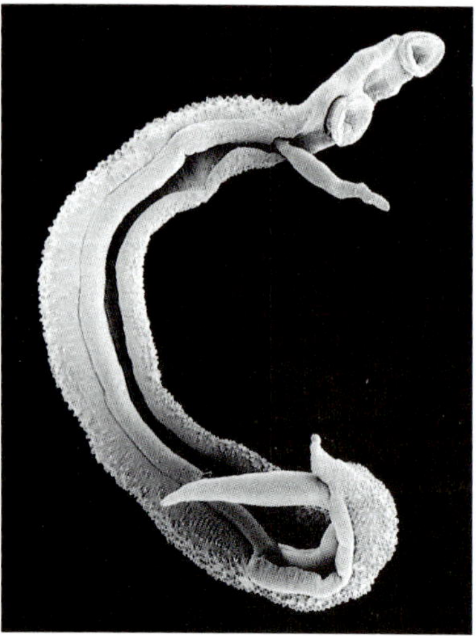

Fig. 3.34 Schistosomiasis. The slender female worm lies in a groove (the gynecophoral canal) in the lateral edge of the body of the male. Scanning electron micrograph. By courtesy of Dr V. Southgate and the publishers of *Systematic Parasitology*.

Schistosome dermatitis is a pruritic papular skin eruption also known as swimmer's itch. It occurs only in individuals who have been previously exposed to schistosome antigens and represents a sensitization reaction. It may occur up to 24 hours after swimming in contaminated water. It is usually caused by infection with avian rather than human schistosomes and thus is common in temperate regions where human schistosomes are not endemic.

Katayama fever is a serum sickness-like syndrome which occurs in heavy infections at the onset of egg deposition. The clinical picture includes fever, chills, sweating, headache, cough, hepatomegaly, splenomegaly, generalized lymphadenopathy and eosinophilia. The symptoms and signs usually disappear within a few weeks but in massive infection due to *S. japonicum* death may occur.

In chronic schistosomiasis there is a progressive increase in the worm burden which affects primarily the intestines (Figs 3.36 & 3.37) and liver (see Fig. 5.30). Chronic granulomatous lesions occur in these organs and may result in portal hypertension, massive splenomegaly and gastrointestinal bleeding from oesophageal varices (Fig. 3.38). The patient experiences fatigue, abdominal pain and diar-

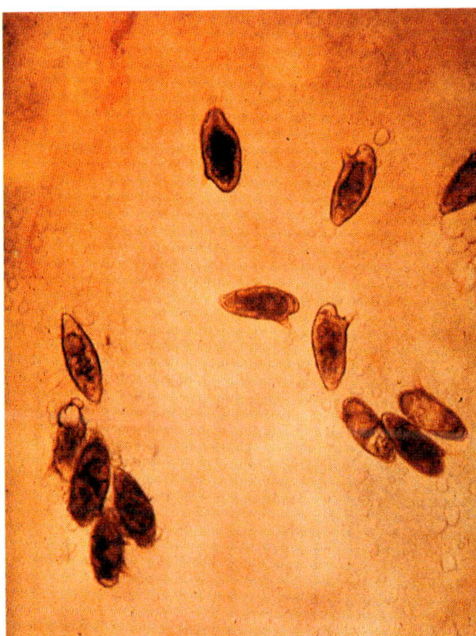

Fig. 3.35 Schistosomiasis. Eggs of *S. mansoni* in faeces showing characteristic lateral spine.

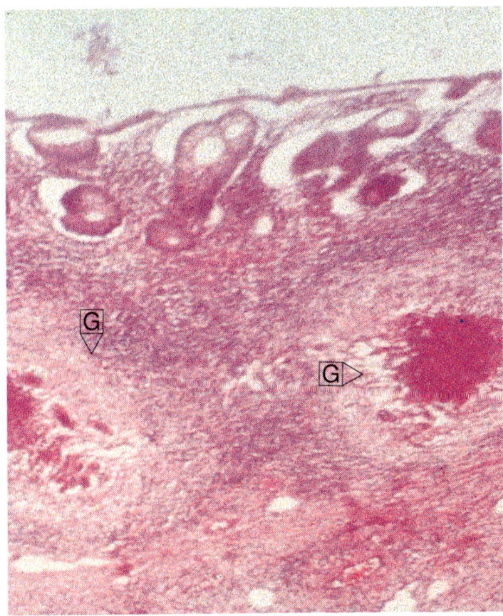

Fig. 3.36 Schistosomiasis. Eggs of *S. mansoni* in mucosa of colon with surrounding granulomatous reaction (G). H&E stain.

rhoea, and in the most severe cases jaundice and liver failure. Occasionally eggs may bypass the liver via the portalsystemic collateral circulation and give rise to granulomas in the lung with pulmonary hypertension and cor pulmonale, or lesions in the brain (Fig. 3.39) or spinal cord which may produce the picture of a space-occupying lesion, generalized encephalopathy or transverse myelitis.

Schistosomiasis is diagnosed by finding the characteristic schistosome eggs in the faeces, in the urine or in a biopsy specimen, usually of the rectal mucosa (see Fig. 3.36). Serological tests have been developed but are not of much practical help in most cases. The development of praziquantel has dramatically improved the effectiveness of drug

therapy of schistosomiasis. Administration of this drug either cures or drastically reduces the worm burden in nearly all cases. The dosage for *S. mansoni* and *S. haematobium* infection is 40 mg/kg, given as a single oral dose; for *S. japonicum* infection the dose is 60 mg/kg given as three doses of 20 mg/kg on one day. Adverse effects are usually mild and include headache, fever and abdominal discomfort.

TAENIASIS

Man is the only definitive host for the beef tapeworm, *Taenia saginata* (Fig. 3.40). Infection occurs when inadequately cooked meat of infected cattle

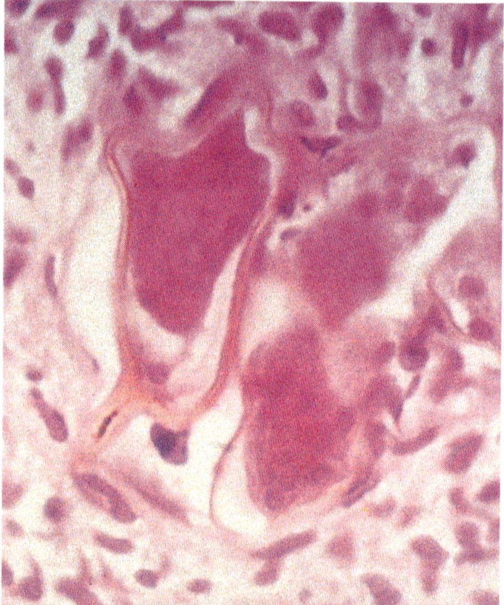

Fig. 3.37 Higher magnification of Fig. 3.36 showing the characteristic lateral spine on one of the eggs. H&E stain.

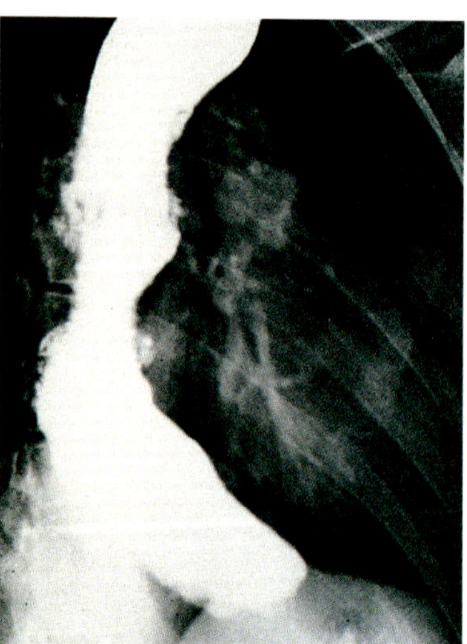

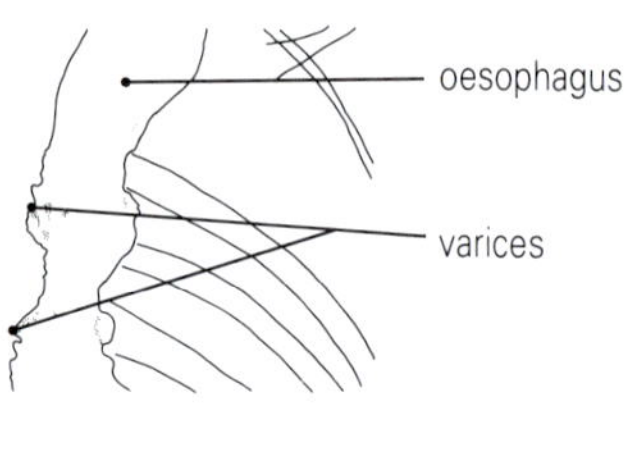

Fig. 3.38 Schistosomiasis. Barium study of oesophagus showing oesophageal varices secondary to portal hypertension in *S. mansoni* infection. By courtesy of Dr I. G. Kagan.

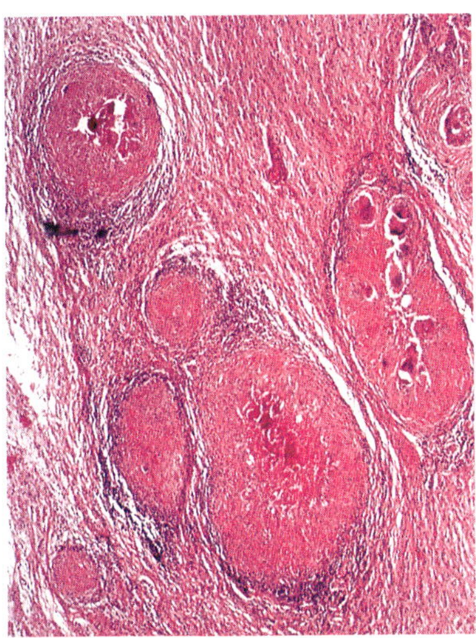

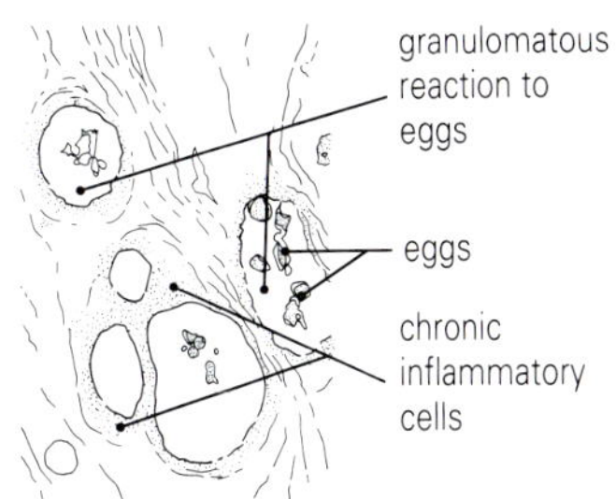

Fig. 3.39 Schistosomiasis. Eggs of *S. japonicum* in gliotic brain with surrounding macrophage and chronic inflammatory cell response. H&E stain.

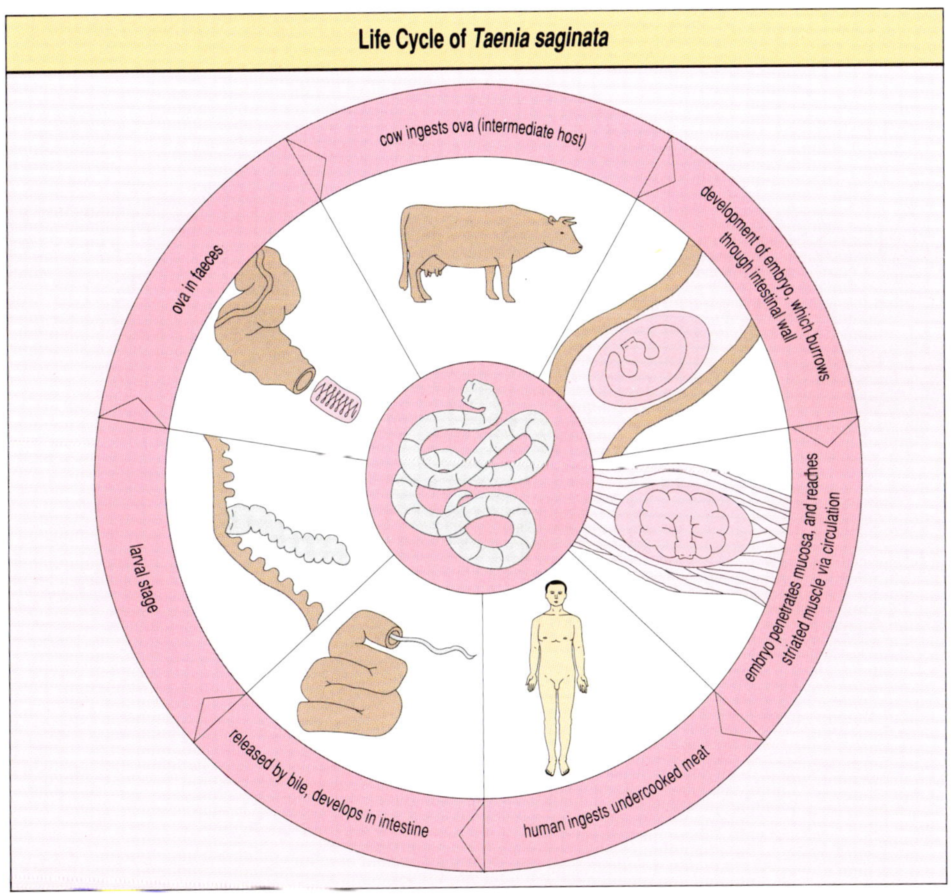

Fig. 3.40 Life cycle of the tapeworm, *Taenia saginata*. A human becomes infected by eating undercooked infected beef. The parasite, released by bile, enters the small intestine where it matures in 2–3 months into a long segmented worm attached to the wall of the intestine by the suckers on its scolex. As segments of the tail mature they are shed into the bowel lumen and escape through the anus. These segments release thousands of eggs, which find their way onto pastures grazed by cattle, especially when sewage is used as fertilizer. If the egg is swallowed by a cow, it develops into an oncosphere, which penetrates the gut wall and enters the circulation. Upon reaching striated muscle it develops into the cysticercus, the infective stage for man. By courtesy of Dr J. Taverne.

is eaten. The encysted larva (cysticercus) in the meat passes through the stomach; in the presence of bile acids in the intestine the larva is released. It attaches to the wall of the intestine and develops into an adult worm, releasing eggs into the lumen of the gut. When these eggs are ingested by cattle the oncospheres penetrate the intestinal wall and the larval forms develop in the muscle tissue. Human tissue does not support growth of the cysticerci, so man is unable to serve as an intermediate host for this organism, although it can serve as an intermediate host for the pork tapeworm, *T. solium* (see below). Infection with *T. saginata* occurs throughout the world. It is most prevalent in Yugoslavia, Moslem countries, Ethiopia and Kenya. It also occurs, albeit less frequently, in Central and South America. Symptoms are usually minimal and consist only of mild abdominal cramps. Rarely a large mass of proglottids causes intestinal or appen-

diceal obstruction. Segments of worm up to several feet in length may be passed per rectum. The only systemic reaction to the worm is mild eosinophilia.

Eggs of *T. saginata* are indistinguishable from those of *T. solium* (Fig. 3.41) but presence of taenia eggs in the faeces should stimulate a search for proglottids (tapeworm segments) by which the two species can be distinguished. Niclosamide (4 tablets chewed thoroughly following a light meal) causes expulsion of the adult worm from the intestine. Paromomycin and praziquantel are also effective. Infection with *T. saginata* can be prevented either by thorough cooking of meat or prevention of human faecal contamination of ground upon which cattle are grazing.

Man can serve as both definitive and intermediate host of the pork tapeworm, *T. solium*. The pathogenesis, symptomatology, diagnosis and treatment of intestinal infection with the adult tape-

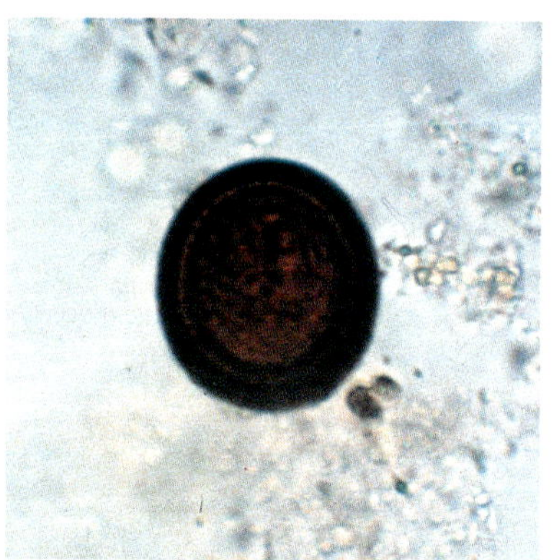

Fig. 3.41 Taeniasis (tapeworm infection). An egg of either *T. solium* or *T. saginata* in faeces containing hexacanth larvae. By courtesy of Dr T.W. Holbrook.

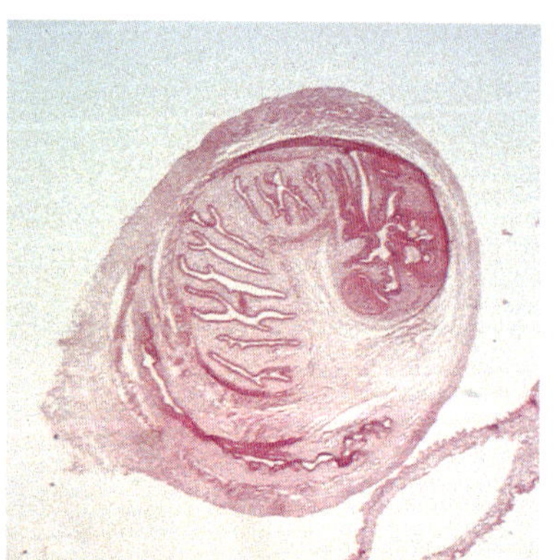

Fig. 3.42 Taeniasis. Scolex of immature *T. solium* in cystic lesion of cysticercosis. H&E stain.

worm are the same as described for *T. saginata*. Man may become the intermediate host for this organism by ingestion of food or water contaminated with infected human faeces, by autoinfection from anus to mouth in an individual already infected with the adult tapeworm and by reverse peristalsis and internal infection. After penetrating the host's intestinal wall the oncosphere develops rapidly and after 10 weeks there is a fully infective larva within the cyst wall (Fig. 3.42). The cysts can develop in almost any part of the body and may produce small mass lesions in the eye, heart, skeletal muscle (Fig. 3.43), skin (Fig. 3.44), or peritoneal cavity. The most important form of cysticercosis is infection of the central nervous system. Both praziquantel and mebendazole are effective in killing the larval stage of the organism, although in many cases the larva has already died and is degenerating at the time symptoms appear.

DIPHYLLOBOTHRIUM LATUM

The adult form of the fish tapeworm *Diphyllobothrium latum* is the largest tapeworm of man, reaching up to 15 metres in length. The eggs released from the gravid proglottids pass out of the body in the faeces and after reaching fresh water, develop into a ciliated oncosphere, the coracidium. This free-swimming form must be eaten within a few days by a copepod (a crustacean), in which it develops into a mature larva called a procercoid. When the copepod is ingested by a fish the procercoid develops into a plerocercoid, or sparganum. If the fish is eaten raw by a mammal the plerocercoid develops after a few weeks into the adult form of *D. latum*.

This infection occurs wherever ingestion of raw fish is common, such as in Scandinavian and Baltic countries, Japan and among Eskimos in Canada

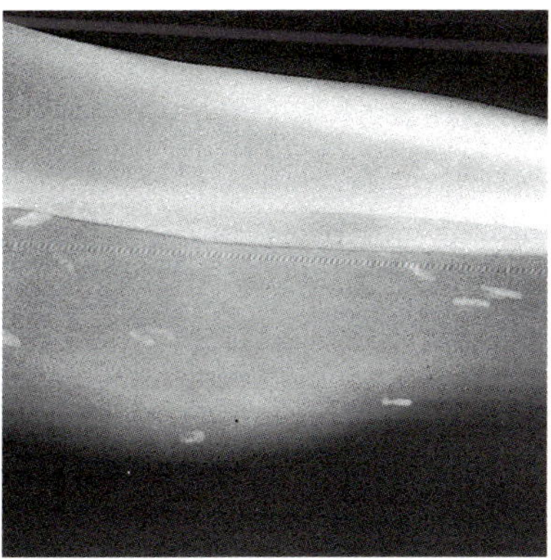

Fig. 3.43 Taeniasis. Radiograph of leg showing characteristic elongated calcified cysts of *T. solium*. At this site they produce no symptoms.

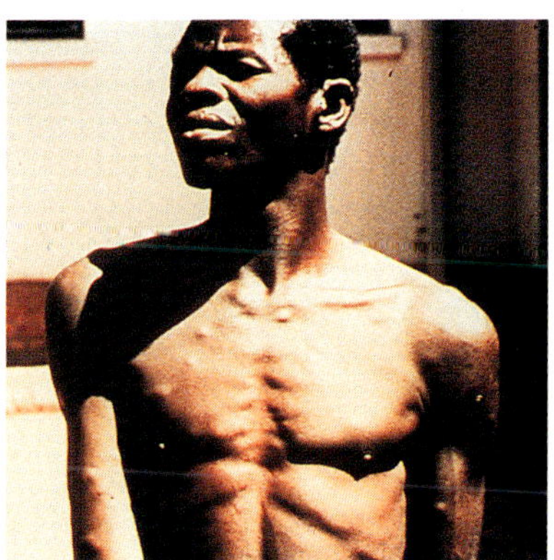

Fig. 3.44 Taeniasis. Infection with the larval form of *T. solium* (cysticercosis) showing multiple subcutaneous cystic lesions containing the larvae, which are known as *Cysticercus cellulosae*. By courtesy of Dr M. G. Schultz.

and Alaska. In the USA, Israel and elsewhere it is seen among Jewish cooks who sample gefilte fish during its preparation.

The symptoms of infection are usually mild but occasionally large masses of the adult worm produce intestinal obstruction. The worm competes with the host for vitamins including vitamin B_{12}; diminished absorption of this vitamin may lead to megaloblastic anaemia or even neurological manifestations of pernicious anaemia, including numbness, paraesthesias, unsteady gait and weakness.

Diagnosis of *D. latum* infection is made by finding the characteristic operculated eggs and proglottids in the faeces. The adult worm may be visualized during barium studies of the upper gastrointestinal tract. Niclosamide, paromomycin and praziquantel are all effective in treatment. Infection with this tapeworm can be prevented by thorough cooking of freshwater fish.

HYMENOLEPIS NANA

Man can serve as both intermediate and definitive host for the dwarf tapeworm, *Hymenolepis nana*. The cycle of internal autoinfection can thus be maintained in a single individual and the infection spread to other humans by faecal contamination of the environment. *H. nana* infection is found throughout the world, but is particularly common in Africa, South America and Eastern Europe. In industrialized countries it is seen most often in children living in crowded institutions. The adult worm is only 25–50 mm in length. Eggs produced by gravid proglottids may either pass out of the body in the faeces or develop into oncospheres which penetrate the villi of the mucosa of the original host. The oncospheres rupture from the villi after approximately 4 days and mature into adult worms in 10–12 days, completing the life cycle. The cycle

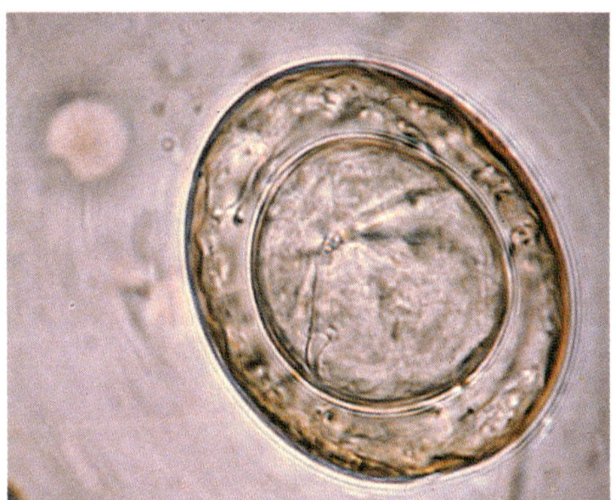

Fig. 3.45 *Hymenolepis nana.* An egg of *H. nana*, with its characteristic double membrane. By courtesy of Dr I. Farrel.

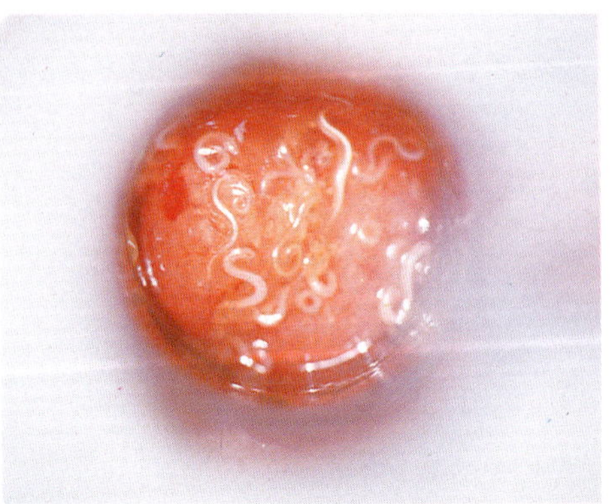

Fig. 3.46 Trichuriasis. Numerous adult *T. trichiura* seen on proctoscopic examination in a healthy infected child. The thin anterior 'whip' end of the worm is secured within the intestinal mucosa, and the thicker posterior end is seen within the lumen. By courtesy of Dr R. H. Gilman.

of internal autoinfection may result in gradually increasing numbers of adult worms in an infected individual. Symptoms of abdominal cramps and diarrhoea may be due to mucosal irritation by adult worms or to rupture of the larvae from the villi. Neurological symptoms of dizziness or seizures may be due to a poorly understood toxin produced by the worms. Diagnosis is made by finding the eggs with their characteristic double membrane in the stools (Fig. 3.45). Treatment with niclosamide should be continued for 5–7 days to eradicate all of the drug-sensitive adult worms as they mature from the drug- resistant cysticercoid stage. Paromomycin and praziquantel are also effective in treatment of this infection.

TRICHURIASIS

Worldwide approximately 500 million people are infected with the whipworm, *Trichuris trichiura*. The infection is most common in tropical areas with poor sanitation facilities. The adult worm inhabits the human caecum and ascending colon. The anterior whiplike portion of the worm is embedded in the wall of the gut while the more robust posterior portion extends into the lumen (Figs 3.46 & 3.47). Eggs are released into the lumen. After excretion in the faeces the embryo develops on moist soil for 2–4 weeks. When the embryonated egg is ingested the larva escapes from the shell and eventually develops into an adult in the caecum or ascending colon.

Most infections are asymptomatic but in a few individuals mild anaemia, bloody diarrhoea and rectal prolapse may develop. Diagnosis is made by finding the characteristic lemon-shaped ova in the faeces (Fig. 3.48). Mebendazole cures or at least drastically reduces the worm burden in nearly all patients.

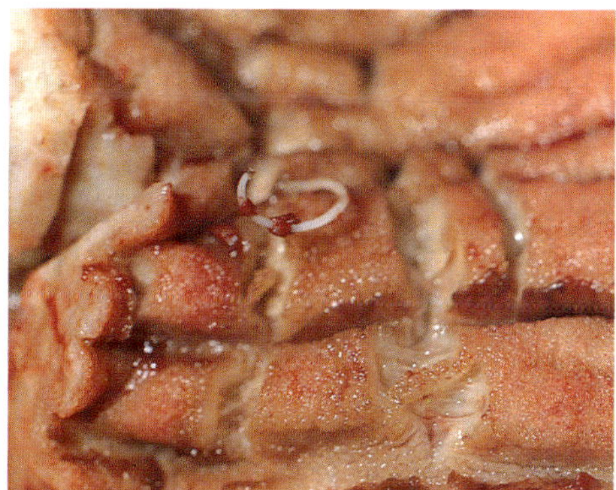

Fig. 3.47 Trichuriasis. A whipworm with its head buried in the ileal mucosa.

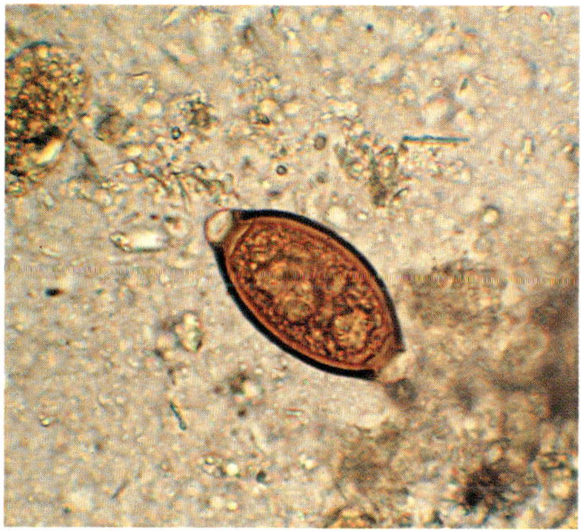

Fig. 3.48 Trichuriasis. Egg of *Trichuris trichiura* in faeces. Note the barrel shape, thick shell and translucent polar prominences.

ENTEROBIASIS

Infection with the pinworm *Enterobius vermicularis* is prevalent throughout the world, especially among school children in temperate regions. It is common at all socio-economic levels, but the highest rates of infection are in crowded populations and among close family of an infected child. The small (10 mm) adult worm inhabits the caecal area and the gravid females migrate at night to the perianal region to release their eggs. The embryonated eggs are transmitted via the hands, night clothes, bedding, air and dust. The lifespan of the adult worm is brief, only about a month, but in highly endemic areas reinfection is common.

Many infections are asymptomatic and in most other infected individuals symptoms are limited to pruritus of the perianal region and perineum, which may interfere with sleep. Rarely migration of the parasite may result in appendicitis (Fig. 3.49), chronic salpingitis or ulcerative lesions of the bowel. Diagnosis is made by examination of a transparent adhesive tape pressed against the perianal region early in the morning (Fig. 3.50). If 5 examinations are done, 99% of infections will be detected. Since the infection rate within families is so high, all members of a family in which a member is found to be infected should be examined. All infected members of the family should receive mebendazole, which has cure rates of 90–100%.

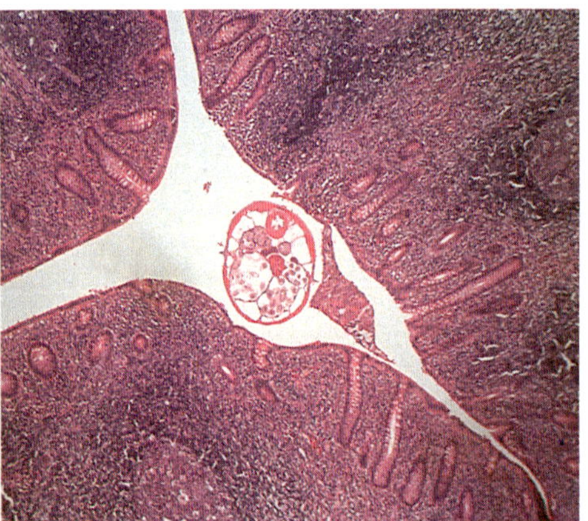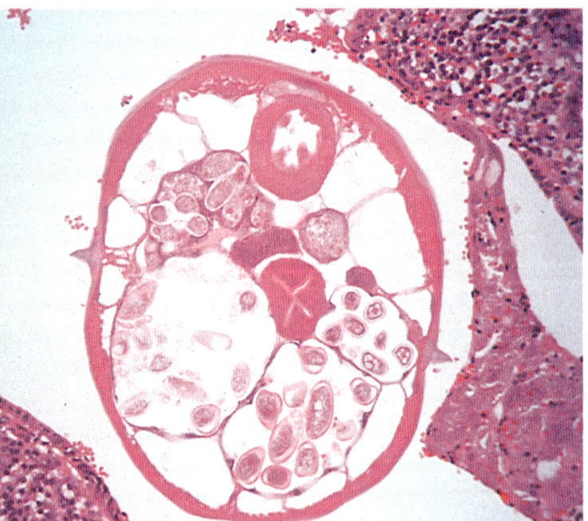

Fig. 3.49 Enterobiasis (pinworm or threadworm infection). Left: Section showing adult pinworm *(Enterobius vermicularis)* in lumen of appendix. Right: Higher magnification, showing numerous eggs within the coiled uteri. H&E stain.

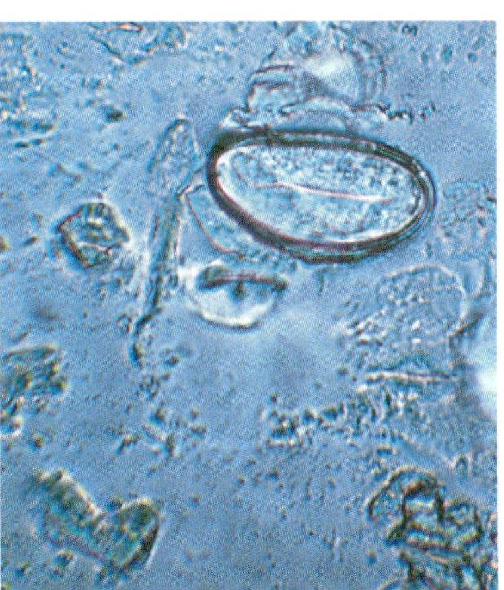

Fig. 3.50 Enterobiasis (pinworm or threadworm infection). A characteristic egg of *E. vermicularis*, collected by adhesive cellophane tape pressed against the perianal area.

ASCARIASIS

Approximately a billion people around the world are infected with the roundworm *Ascaris lumbricoides* (Fig. 3.51). Although this organism is worldwide in distribution, infection is most prevalent in tropical countries. The adult worm, 15–35 cm in length (Figs 3.52 & 3.53), normally inhabits the lumen of the jejunum and middle ileum. Each female worm produces an enormous number of eggs, approximately 200 000 per day. These are passed from the body in the faeces and, under warm moist conditions, develop into mature infective embryos within 10 days. After ingestion they hatch in the small intestine; the embryos penetrate the wall of the gut and migrate through the venous

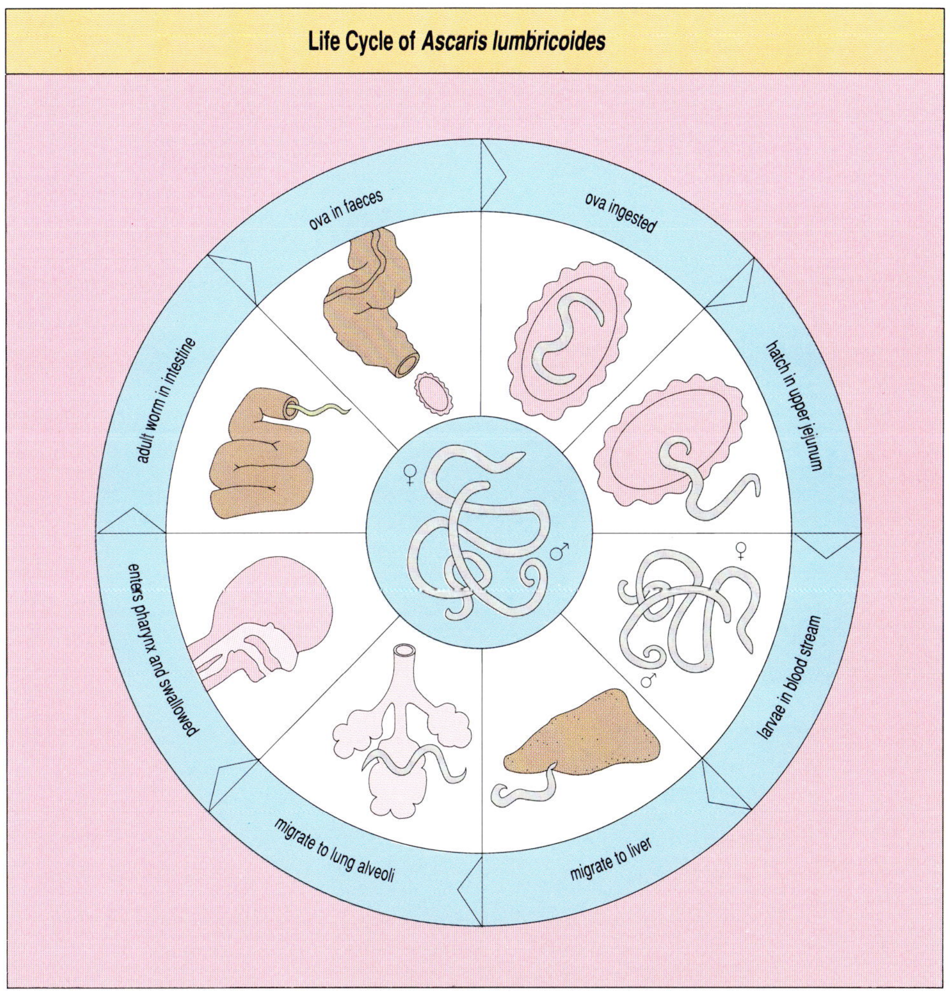

Fig. 3.51 Life cycle of *Ascaris lumbricoides*. *A. lumbricoides* is transmitted to man directly from the soil, without the mediation of a vector. Following ingestion of the ova, the larvae hatch in the small intestine and are carried in the bloodstream to the liver, from where they migrate to the lungs. They then pass through the trachea, throat and oesophagus, and return to the intestine where they mature in 2–3 months into adult worms. The adult worms live in the intestinal lumen for 12–18 months, so infection does not persist in the absence of re-exposure. Eggs pass out in the faeces at the single cell stage. The eggs may survive in the soil for months or even years. If the temperature and humidity are suitable, they develop into active embryos and can become fully infective within 2–3 weeks. By courtesy of Dr J. Taverne.

system to the heart and lungs (Figs 3.54 & 3.55) where they break out into the alveoli, pass up through the bronchial system and are swallowed, finally reaching the intestine to develop into mature worms. Most infections are asymptomatic, but heavy infection can interfere with intestinal absorption and lead to malnutrition. Rarely a mass of worms (Fig. 3.56) may obstruct the lumen of the small bowel and produce an acute illness with vomiting, abdominal distension and cramping pain. During such an attack worms may be passed in vomitus or in stools. A worm may invade the common bile duct, producing obstruction with colicky abdominal pain, nausea and vomiting (Figs 3.57 & 3.58). When large numbers of larvae migrate through the lungs in an individual who is sensitized to ascaris antigens, an allergic pneumonitis resembling Löffler's syndrome may result, with respiratory symptoms and eosinophilia in the peripheral blood.

The diagnosis can be made by finding the unfertilized or embryonated eggs on direct examination

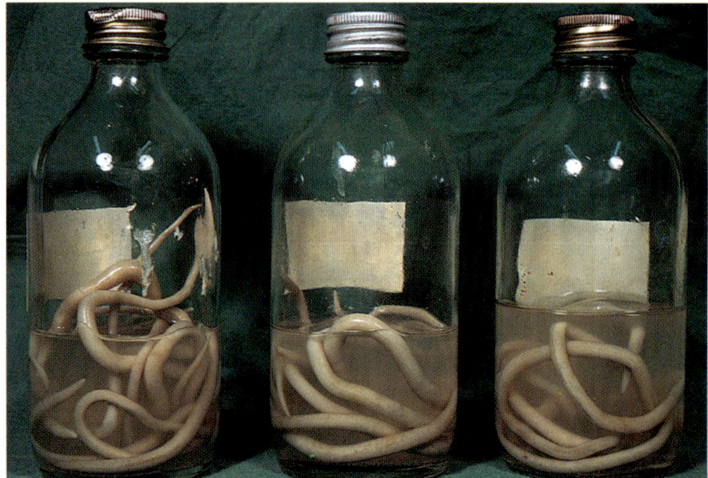

Fig. 3.52 Ascariasis. Large adult worms of *Ascaris lumbricoides*.

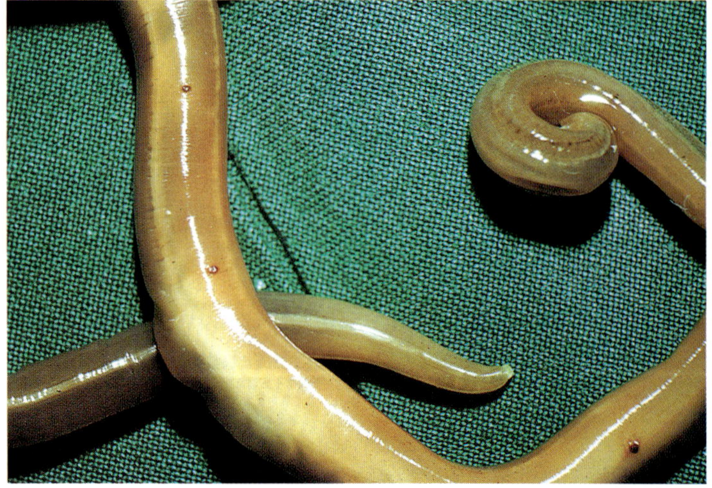

Fig. 3.53 Ascariasis. Large adult worms of *Ascaris lumbricoides*.

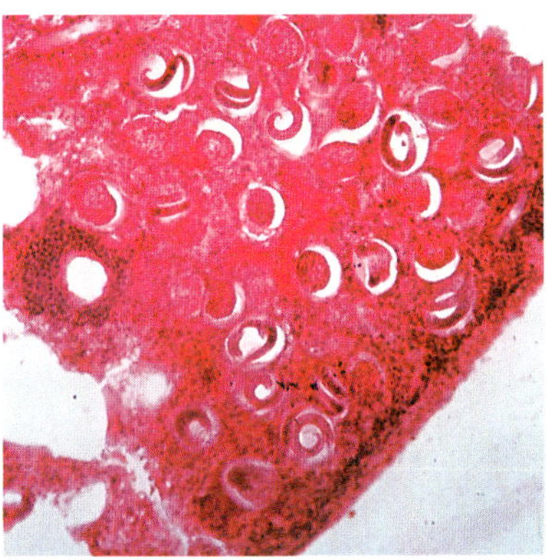

Fig. 3.54 Ascariasis. Section of lung showing very heavy infection with larvae of *A. lumbricoides*. H&E stain.

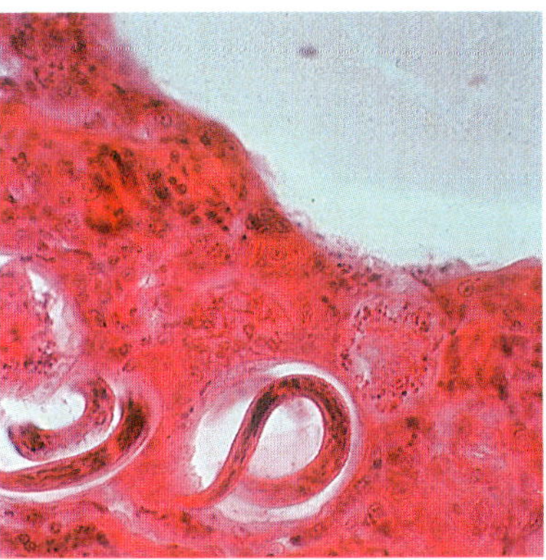

Fig. 3.55 Ascariasis. Higher magnification of Fig. 3.54 showing detail of larva and surrounding inflammatory reaction. H&E stain.

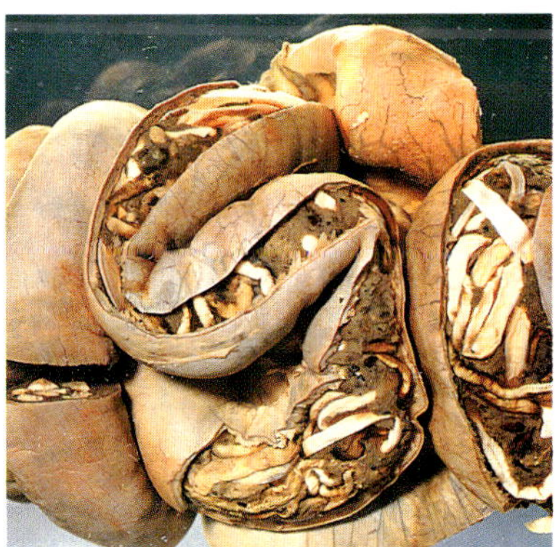

Fig. 3.56 Bolus of ascaris worms in the gut causing intestinal obstruction. By courtesy of Dr D. R. Davies.

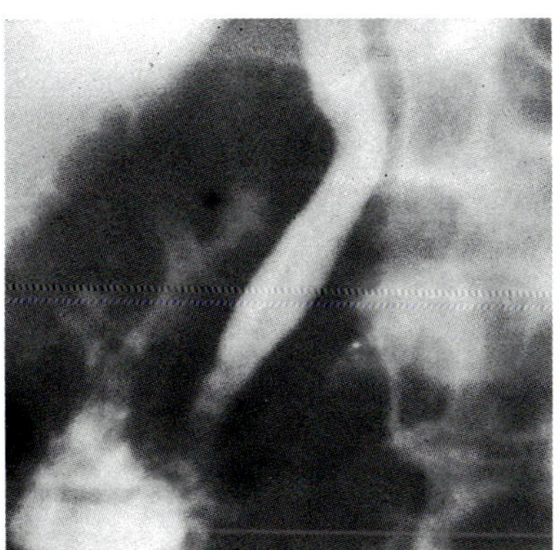

Fig. 3.57 Ascariasis. A single *A. lumbricoides* is visible within the common bile duct. Contrast material can also be seen in the alimentary tract of the worm, which was subsequently removed by sphincterotomy. By courtesy of Dr J. Cunningham.

of a stool specimen (Figs 3.59, 3.60 & 3.61). Occasionally an adult worm is seen during barium examination of the small intestine (Figs 3.62 & 3.63). The most effective treatment for intestinal infection with *A. lumbricoides* is mebendazole. If intestinal or biliary obstruction is suspected, piperazine citrate should be used, as this drug narcotizes the worms and prevents further aggravation of the obstruction.

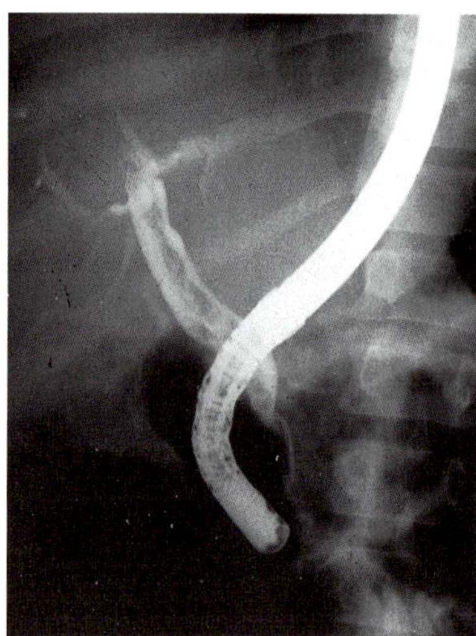

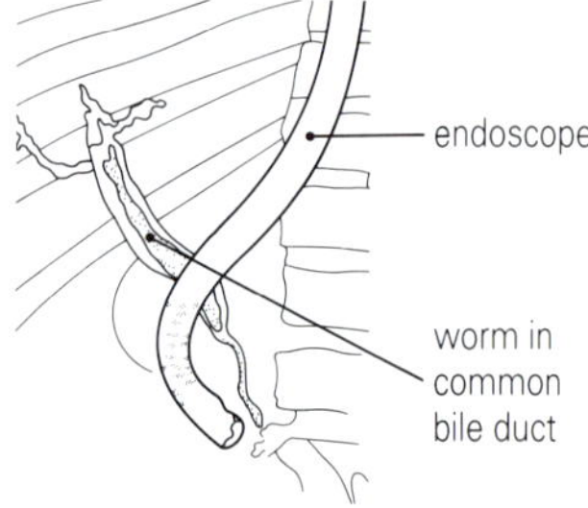

Fig. 3.58 ERCP showing an ascaris worm in the common bile duct of a young African patient presenting with acute pancreatitis and cholangitis. By courtesy of Dr A. Hatfield.

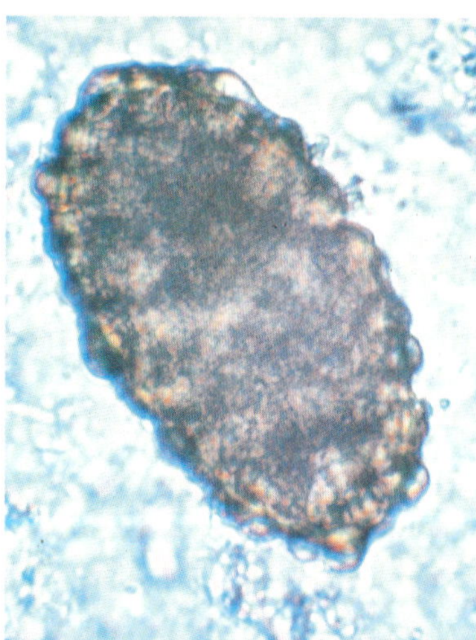

Fig. 3.59 Ascariasis. Unfertilized egg of *A. lumbricoides* in faeces showing pronounced ellipsoidal shape and indistinct internal structure. This type of egg may be seen in patients harbouring only female worms and they are occasionally mistaken for vegetable cells.

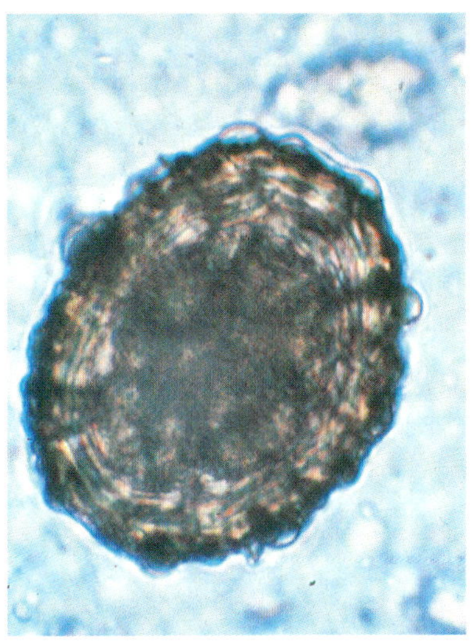

Fig. 3.60 Ascariasis. Fertilized egg of *A. lumbricoides* in faeces showing more rounded shape and corticated outer shell.

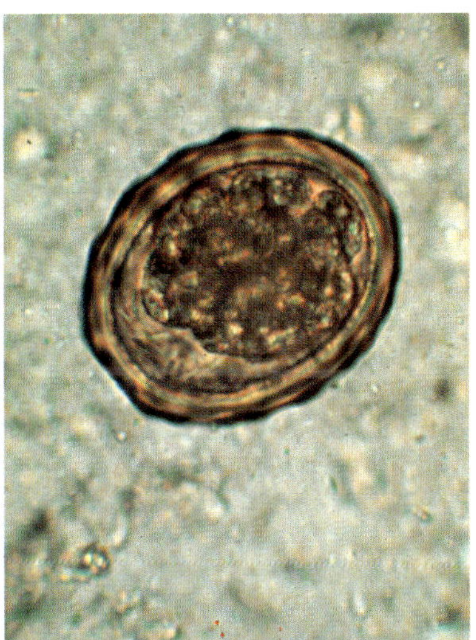

Fig. 3.61 Ascariasis. Embryonated egg of *A. lumbricoides* containing more mature embryo and showing less pronounced cortication of outer shell.

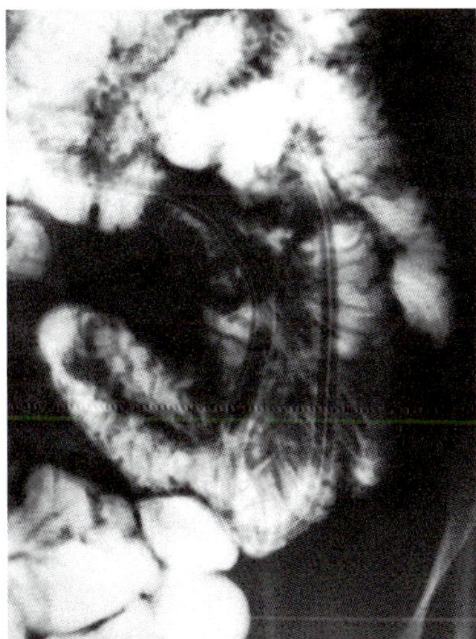

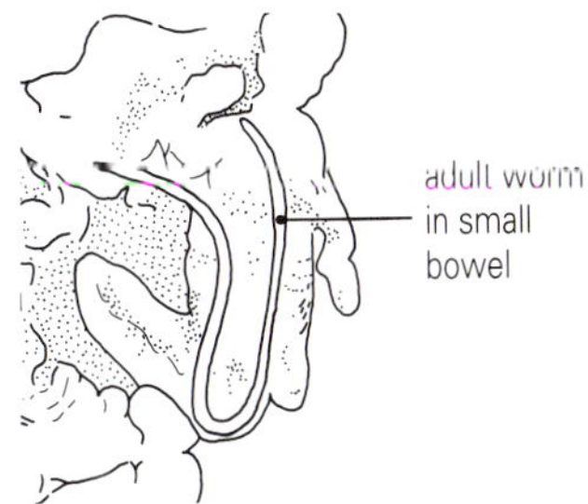

Fig. 3.62 Ascariasis. Barium study of small bowel in a patient with ascariasis. The intestinal tract of one of the adult worms is also well-outlined with barium which it has ingested.

HOOKWORM

Infection with one of the two species of hookworm, *Necator americanus* and *Ancylostoma duodenale,* affects approximately one billion individuals, mainly in tropical and subtropical regions. The adults are small (10 mm), cylindrical worms which live attached to the mucosa of the upper small intestine by means of their buccal capsules (Fig. 3.64). The eggs pass out of the body with the stools and under suitable conditions of temperature and humidity hatch into larvae which can penetrate intact human skin. They are carried through the venous system to the lungs where they penetrate the alveolar walls, make their way up the trachea and are swallowed, to reach their final habitat in the small intestine. Efficient transmission thus depends on two factors: the disposal of human faecal waste on the ground, and the habit of walking barefoot.

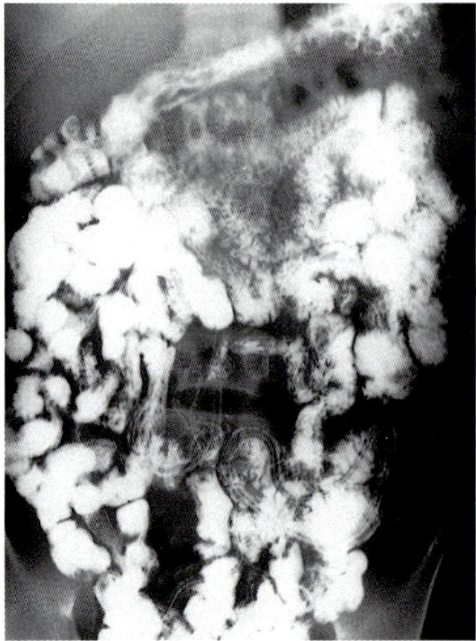

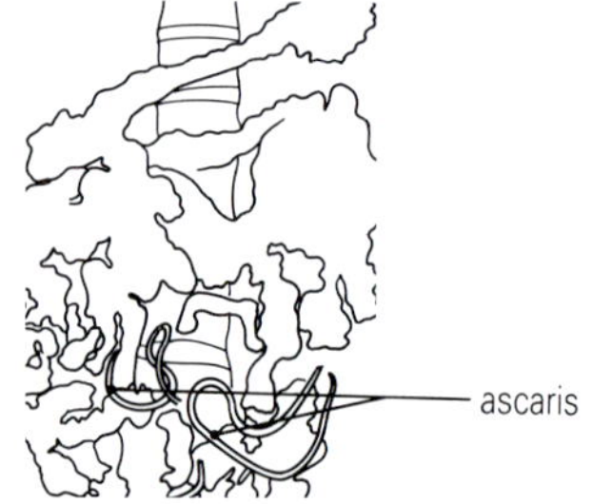

Fig. 3.63 Barium study showing ascaris in the small intestine.

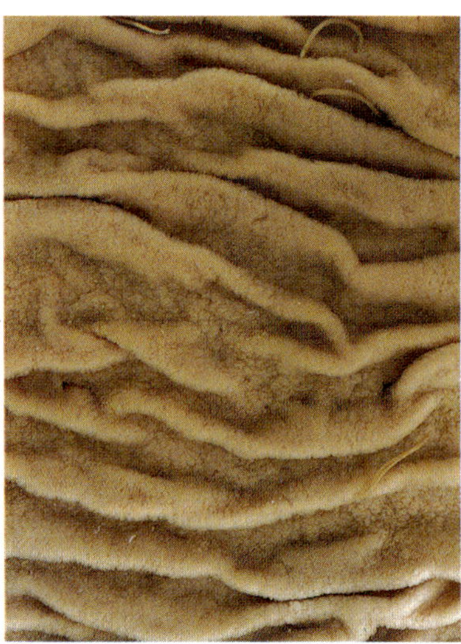

Fig. 3.64 Hookworm infection. A short section of infected intestine. By courtesy of Dr D. R. Davies.

Iron deficiency anaemia and hypoalbuminaemia due to intestinal blood loss are the major clinical manifestations of hookworm infection. 'Ground itch', (an intense pruritus, erythema and papulovesicular rash) may result from the penetration of larvae through the skin. As the larvae migrate through the lungs, a Löffler–like syndrome may occur with cough, wheezing and sputum production, with infiltrates on the chest x-ray and eosinophilia in the sputum and peripheral blood.

In heavy infections abdominal pain, diarrhoea and weight loss may occur.

The diagnosis is made by finding the eggs in the faeces. The two species cannot be distinguished by the appearance of the eggs. In freshly-passed stool specimens the eggs seen are non-embryonated (Fig. 3.65), but if the specimen has been at room temperature for several hours, embryos of various stages may be seen within the eggs (Figs 3.66 & 3.67). Because of the potential for production of

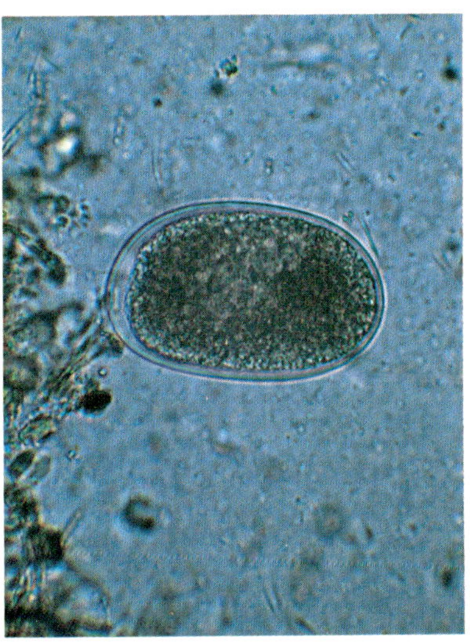

Fig. 3.65 Hookworm infection. Non-embryonated egg of *Necator americanus* in a freshly-passed stool specimen. (Eggs of *N. americanus* and *Ancylostoma duodenale* are difficult to distinguish from one another, although adults can be differentiated easily.)

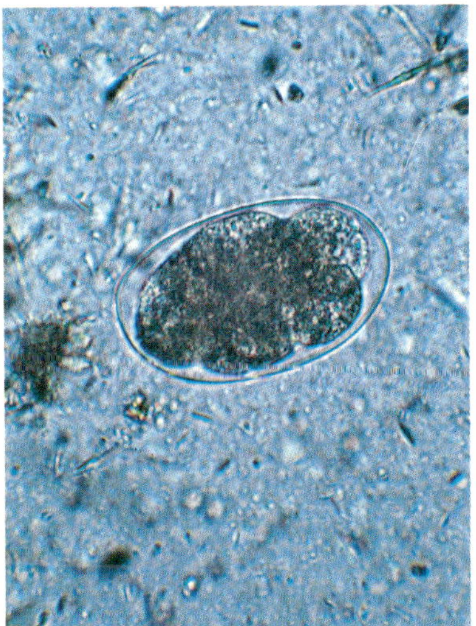

Fig. 3.66 Hookworm infection. Embryonated egg of *N. americanus* in which cell division has begun.

significant clinical illness, heavy hookworm infection should be treated with mebendazole. The anaemia should be treated with iron.

STRONGYLOIDIASIS

Infection with the nematode *Strongyloides stercoralis* is uncommon in comparison with the nematode infections discussed above, but is nontheless widely distributed in tropical countries. The prevalence of infection may be as high as 4% in some southern states of the USA. The adult worms inhabit the upper small intestine where the females burrow through the mucosa, depositing ova in the tissues (Figs 3.68 & 3.69). The larvae hatch in the mucosa and bore through the epithelium into the lumen, where they are normally passed in the faeces (Fig. 3.70). After leaving the body they may develop into

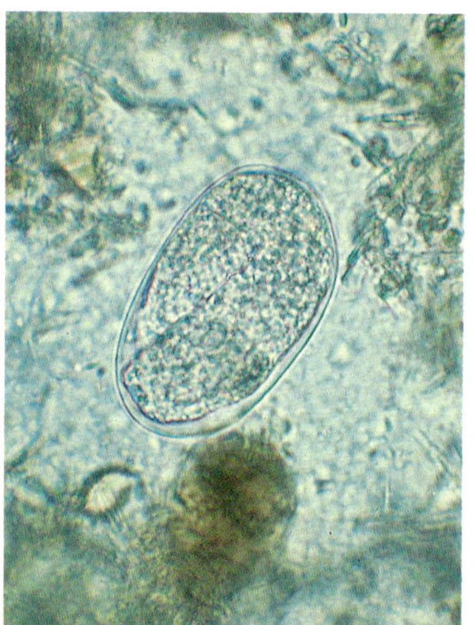

Fig. 3.67 Hookworm infection. Egg of *N. americanus* in faeces containing a relatively mature embryo.

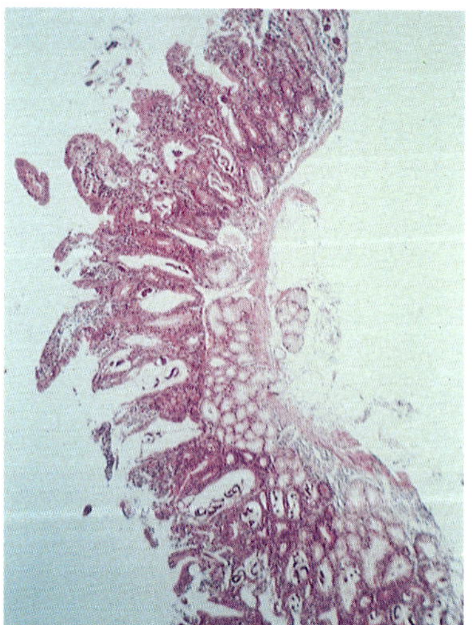

Fig. 3.68 Strongyloidiasis. Section of duodenal mucosa showing the very small adult worms of *Strongyloides stercoralis* in the crypts of the mucosa. H&E stain.

either free-living adults or infective filariform larvae. If the latter come into contact with human skin, they may penetrate it, pass by way of the venous system to the lungs, ascend to the glottis where they are swallowed and finally reach the small intestine. Some larvae may develop into filariform worms in the lumen of the gut and penetrate the intestinal mucosa of the individual in which they originated.

A pruritic skin rash may be produced at the site of penetration of the larvae through the skin. A pneumonitis resembling Löffler's syndrome can occur as the larvae migrate through the lungs. Invasion of the intestinal mucosa by the organisms may produce colicky abdominal pain, diarrhoea, nausea, vomiting and weight loss. Eosinophilia is usually present. Autoinfection may result in massive larval invasion of the lungs and other organs, particularly

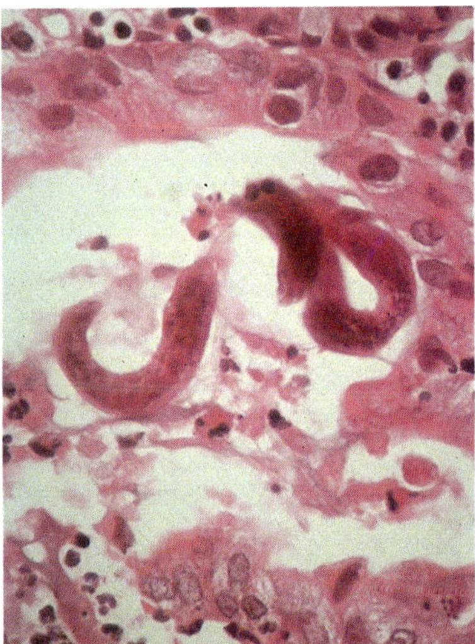

Fig. 3.69 Stronglyloidiasis. Higher magnification showing adult *S. stercoralis* in crypt in jejunal mucosa. H&E stain.

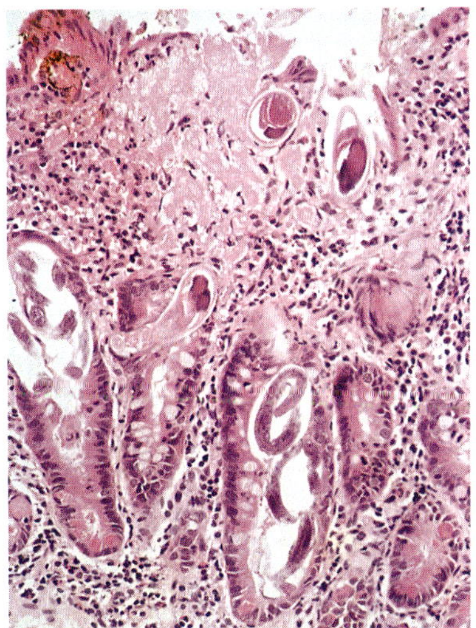

Fig. 3.70 Stronglyloides. Ulcerated jejunal mucosa showing adult and larval forms of *Strongyloides stercoralis*. No eggs are visible here. ×120. H&E stain.

in immunocompromised hosts (Fig. 3.71). This type of disseminated infection has been described following chemotherapy for lymphomas and leukaemias, in patients with lepromatous leprosy and in individuals treated with corticosteroids. Treatment with corticosteroids may suppress the eosinophilia which is usually observed in these patients. Patients with overwhelming autoinfection may exhibit severe generalized abdominal pain, diffuse pulmonary infiltrates, ileus, shock and meningitis or sepsis from gram-negative bacilli. Recurrent meningitis due to intestinal bacteria has been reported in a few cases.

The diagnosis is made by demonstrating the larvae of *S. stercoralis* in the faeces or duodenal fluid (Figs 3.72 & 3.73). Concentration of the specimen by the zinc sulphate method may be necessary. Duodenal contents may be sampled by the Enterotest technique used in the diagnosis of *Giardia lamblia* infection. The only drug effective in

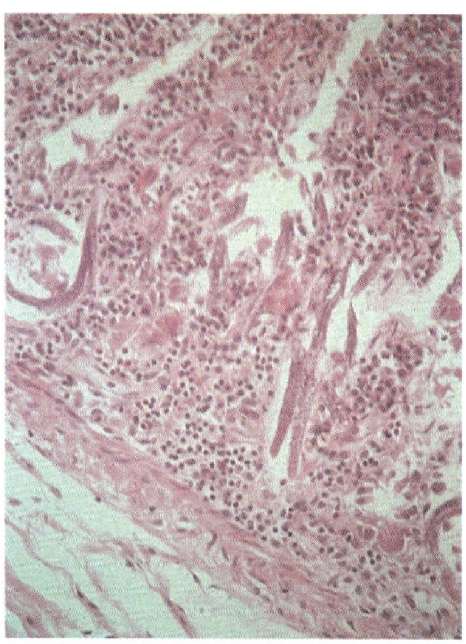

Fig. 3.71 Strongyloidiasis. Massive invasion of a lymph node by larvae of *S. stercoralis* in disseminated infection in an immunocompromised patient. H&E stain.

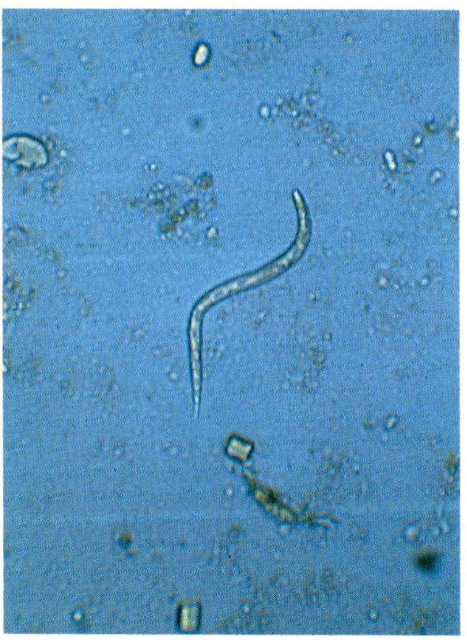

Fig. 3.72 Strongyloidiasis. Rhabditiform larva of *S. stercoralis* in faeces. At this magnification it is very difficult to distinguish from the larvae of hookworms.×100.

the treatment of *S. stercoralis* infection is thiabendazole. In the hyperinfection syndrome treatment should be continued for 2–3 weeks.

Viral Infections

Acute viral gastroenteritis is a major global cause of serious morbidity, especially in infants and young children, in whom diarrhoea and vomiting may rapidly lead to malnutrition, dehydration and serious electrolyte imbalance (Fig. 3.74). Acute gastroenteritis affects approximately 500 million children per year worldwide. In less developed countries it is the leading cause of death in children under the age of 4 years. In developed countries viral gastroenteritis is second in prevalence only to viral upper respiratory tract illness. During the last 20 years a number of viruses associated with acute gastroenteritis have been identified. These include the rotaviruses, fastidious faecal adenoviruses, Norwalk virus and Norwalk-like agents, caliciviruses, astroviruses and coronaviruses.

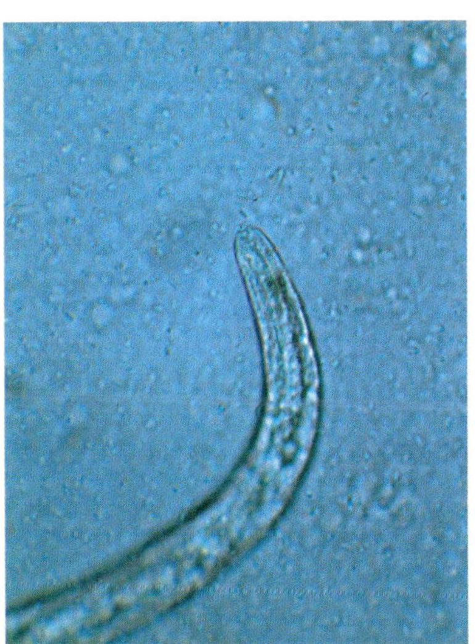

Fig. 3.73 Strongyloidiasis. Higher magnification of rhabditiform larva of *S. stercoralis* showing the short buccal capsule. Larvae of hookworms have a much longer buccal capsule. ×400.

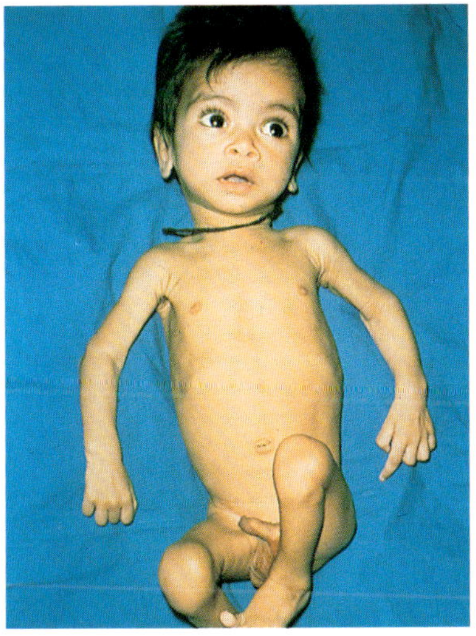

Fig. 3.74 Viral gastroenteritis. Note the alert expression, flaccid posture and general appearance of dehydration and malnutrition.

ROTAVIRUSES

Rotaviruses are members of the family *Reoviridae.* They possess a double layer of icosahedral shells approximately 70 nm in diameter, and have a core of double-stranded RNA (Fig. 3.75). They have been classified into a number of different types based on the electrophoretic mobility of the 11 different segments of the RNA genome. Segments which exhibit similar electrophoretic mobility do not necessarily exhibit RNA homology, but the electrophoretic patterns are useful in epidemiological studies. At least 4 and possibly as many as 6 serotypes of human rotaviruses have also been identified.

Diarrhoeal disease due to rotaviruses most commonly affects young children. Infected neonates are often asymptomatic and the parents of infected children may exhibit only a rise in serum antibody titres. Rotaviruses are prevalent in day-care centres, where they are readily transmitted by the faecal–oral route to other children and to family contacts. The illness may be relatively severe in the elderly, and fatal infections have occurred in individuals living in nursing homes. Rotaviruses are responsible for approximately 50% of all cases of paediatric gastroenteritis requiring hospitalization in the world's temperate zones. The two most common features of rotavirus disease are diarrhoea and vomiting. The vomiting

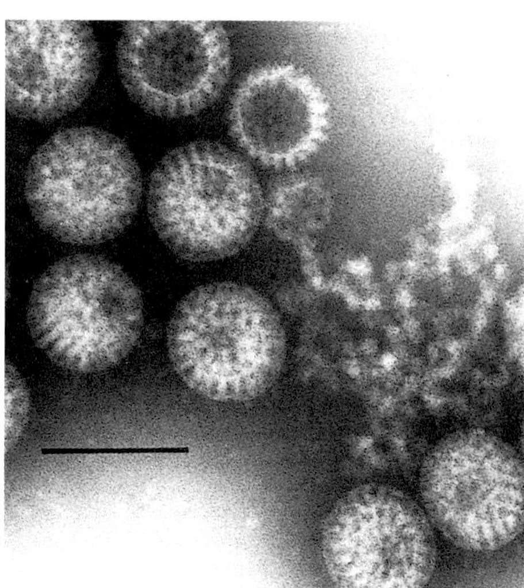

Fig. 3.75 Rotavirus. Electron micrograph showing negatively-stained particles approximately 75 nm in diameter in faeces. The 'spoked-wheel' appearance is characteristic. Bar = 100 nm. By courtesy of Regional Virus Laboratory, East Birmingham Hospital, Birmingham, England.

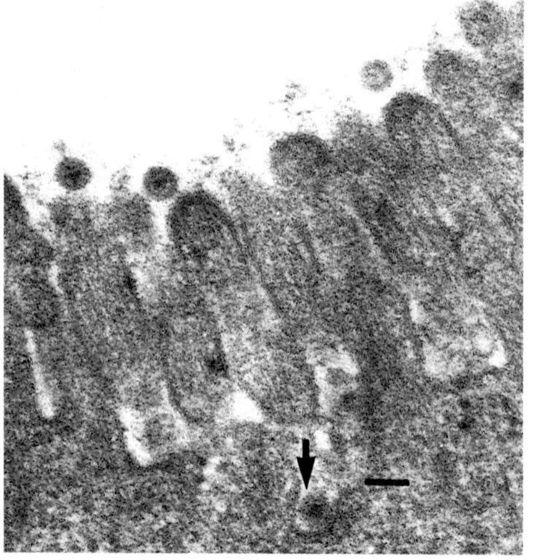

Fig. 3.76 Rotavirus. Electron micrograph showing thin section of enterocyte with heavy infective load of rotaviruses. One has penetrated the brush border. Bar = 100 nm. By courtesy of Dr K. Coehlo.

often precedes the diarrhoea. It is not known for certain whether rotaviruses cause respiratory symptoms. The diarrhoea often lasts 5–8 days and, in small children, often results in dehydration and electrolyte imbalance.

Rotaviruses primarily affect the small intestine; virus replication takes place in epithelial cells at the tips of the villi. The patchy mucosal changes include shortening and blunting of the villi and increased infiltration of the lamina propria with mononuclear cells. The epithelial cells become more cuboidal and less regular than normal. Reovirus-like particles may be seen by electron microscopy in the epithelial cells of the duodenal mucosa (Fig. 3.76). Functionally, low levels of activity of maltase, sucrase and lactase occur; these abnormalities return to normal after 4–8 weeks. Most children exhibit malabsorption of lactose and lactose intolerance; an increase in the diarrhoea may occur after ingestion of lactose.

Large amounts of rotavirus are excreted in the stool during acute gastroenteritis and the virus can be seen upon direct examination of the stool by electron microscopy (EM) (see Fig. 3.75). Immune electron microscopy (IEM), in which the faecal suspension is mixed with specific antiserum, is even more sensitive than direct examination. However, electron microscopic procedures are time consuming and expensive, so most laboratories employ the enzyme-linked immunosorbent assay (ELISA) or latex agglutination (LA) tests, for which several commercial kits are available.

The mechanisms involved in protection and recovery from rotavirus infection are complex and appear to involve both local and systemic humoral and cell-mediated responses and also possibly other non-specific factors. Vaccine development has concentrated on oral vaccines which stimulate production of local intestinal IgA antibody. Vaccines utilizing attenuated strains of both bovine and monkey rotaviruses, as well as reassortant vaccines, are under investigation.

Treatment of rotavirus infections (and of other diarrhoeal diseases due to viruses) is based on the replacement of water and electrolytes in dehydrated patients. Although a few patients require initial therapy with intravenous fluids, by far the great majority of patients can be treated with oral replacement solutions. These solutions contain both electrolytes and glucose; the latter is required for glucose-coupled sodium transport in the small intestine. After dehydration and electrolyte imbalance are corrected, feedings begin with breast milk or dilute formula and progress to full-strength formula over two or three days. Bland carbohydrate solid foods which do not contain lactose, such as rice, cereal and potatoes, are reintroduced as soon as tolerated.

ADENOVIRUSES

Adenoviruses are probably second only to rotaviruses in importance as viral causes of diarrhoeal disease (Fig. 3.77). These are 70–75 nm, non-

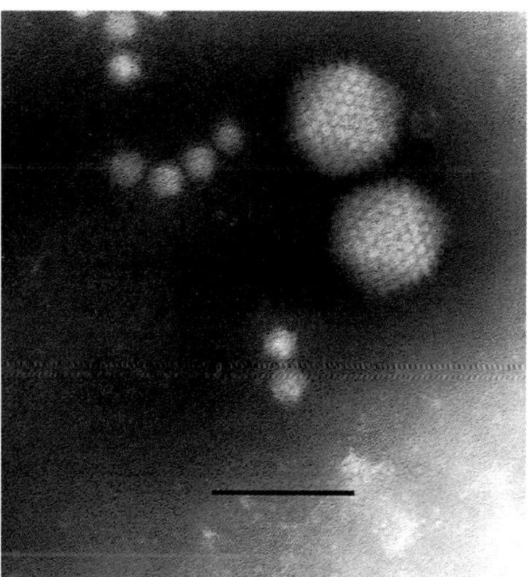

Fig. 3.77 Adenovirus. Electron micrograph showing negatively-stained particles of approximately 80 nm diameter, isolated from faeces. Note the typical hexagonal outline produced by the icosahedral structure. The very small particles are adeno-associated (satellite) viruses. Bar = 100nm. By courtesy of Regional Virus Laboratory, East Birmingham Hospital Birmingham, England.

enveloped, icosahedral, double stranded DNA viruses which infect many species of mammals and lower animals. Of the 41 serotypes which infect man, types 40 and 41 are designated 'fastidious' adenoviruses, as they cannot be isolated in routine cell cultures and exhibit DNA restriction patterns which differ from those of the other serotypes. Although non-fastidious respiratory adenoviruses may cause diarrhoeal disease in humans, the fastidious adenoviruses appear to be more important causes of viral gastroenteritis. Whether or not these agents can also cause respiratory disease is unknown. Fastidious adenoviruses cause infection and disease primarily in children under the age of 2 years.

Diarrhoea with or without vomiting is the predominant symptom. Severity may range from a mild afebrile illness to a severe or even fatal disease with profound dehydration. Most patients infected with adenoviruses have milder disease with less pronounced vomiting, less fever and less diarrhoea than patients infected with rotaviruses. Respiratory symptoms are more common in patients infected with adenoviruses.

Type-specific ELISA using monoclonal antibodies to the fastidious types 40 and 41 have been developed, but these tests are not in routine clinical use at the present time.

NORWALK VIRUS AND NORWALK-LIKE AGENTS

Norwalk virus is a small round virus, 25–30 nm in diameter, which cannot be cultivated *in vitro*. A number of other Norwalk-like viruses, some of which are antigenically similar to Norwalk virus, have also been found in association with outbreaks of acute non-bacterial gastroenteritis (Fig. 3.78). Transmission apparently occurs via ingestion of contaminated water or food or by person-to-person spread. In industrialized countries Norwalk and similar viruses tend to infect older children and adults, suggesting that exposure to these viruses is uncommon during early childhood. In the USA and Canada, antibody to Norwalk virus is found in only 5% of children up to the age of 12 years, but prevalence of antibody increases rapidly during adolescence and young adulthood. In less developed countries antibody usually appears during childhood.

The incubation period is usually 24–48 hours. Onset of illness is sudden with nausea and vomit-

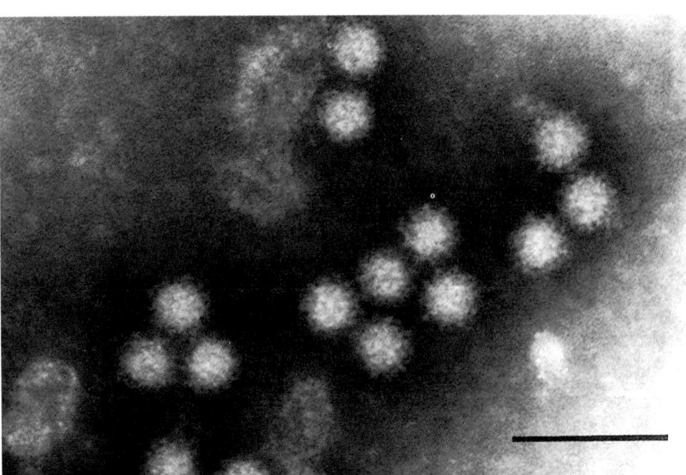

Fig. 3.78 Small round structured virus (similar morphology to Norwalk agent). Electron micrograph showing negatively-stained particles of 33–38nm diameter. These particles show little organized surface structure, but the appearance is consistent. Bar = 100 nm. By courtesy of Regional Virus Laboratory, East Birmingham Hospital Birmingham, England.

ing, which is often severe, low-grade fever and diarrhoea, which may be mild. Other symptoms include mild abdominal pain or cramps, headache and malaise. The attack rate in outbreaks may be as high as 50%. Respiratory symptoms apparently do not occur as a result of infection with Norwalk or similar viruses. In children vomiting is usually the predominant symptom, whereas adults are more likely to experience diarrhoea. Hospitalization is rarely required, but a few cases of serious illness have been reported. Intestinal mucosal biopsy has revealed mild changes similar to those seen in gastroenteritis due to other viruses, and transient deficiency in intestinal enzyme activity may occur.

Only small numbers of Norwalk and similar viruses are present in the faeces in infected individuals, so the agent can rarely be detected by direct EM. Clumps of viral particles can often be visualized by the more sensitive technique of IEM. Radioimmunoassays and ELISAs have been developed and utilized in epidemiological studies, but are rarely available in clinical microbiology laboratories.

Immunity to Norwalk virus appears to be complex. Most volunteers given Norwalk virus who become ill have pre-existing Norwalk antibody, whereas the majority of volunteers who do not become ill have little or no pre-existing antibody in the serum. Protective mechanisms other than serum antibody must be important.

OTHER VIRAL CAUSES OF ACUTE GASTROENTERITIS

Three other groups of viruses, the caliciviruses, astroviruses and coronaviruses, have been implicated in acute gastroenteritis in humans.

Caliciviruses are small RNA viruses, approximately 30 nm in diameter. There are 32 cup-shaped depressions on the surface of the virion, which gives the particle a spiky appearance and a six-pointed Star of David configuration at certain orientations. These viruses cause gastroenteritis primarily in infants and young children. In most areas of the world a majority of individuals exhibit antibody to caliciviruses by the age of 5 years. The symptoms of calicivirus infection are similar to those of rotavirus infection. Diarrhoea is usually the predominant feature, but in some studies vomiting has also been common. Upper respiratory tract symptoms and fever occur in a significant minority of patients. Caliciviruses may be seen in the stools by direct EM and IEM (Fig. 3.79), but cannot be isolated in routine cell cultures.

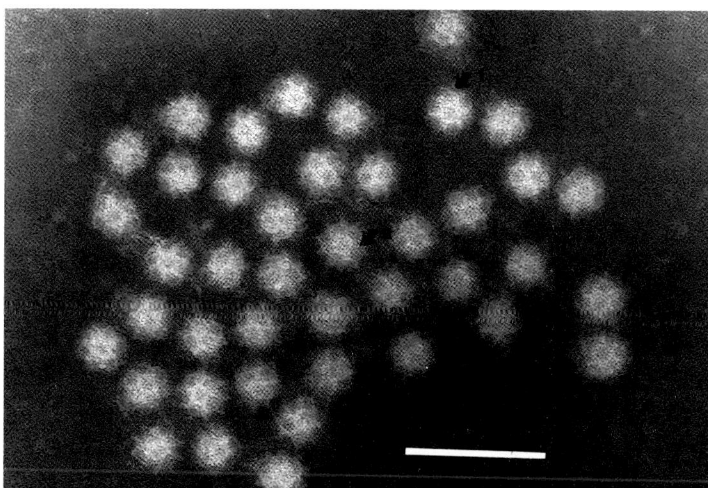

Fig. 3.79 Calicivirus. Electron micrograph showing negatively-stained particles of 33–38 nm diameter in faeces. A characteristic appearance is the 6-pointed star of David with a central hole. Also shown is a 10-pointed sphere. Bar = 100 nm. By courtesy of Regional Virus Laboratory, East Birmingham Hospital Birmingham, England.

Astroviruses are 28–30 nm round virus particles which have a smooth edge. The particles may have either a 5- or 6-point star-like configuration. These viruses may be detected in stool suspensions by direct EM (Fig. 3.80) and also can be propagated in HEK cells. There are at least five distinct serotypes of human astroviruses. Children from infancy up to the age of 7 years are most often affected. Symptomatic children have watery diarrhoea, vomiting or both. The illness is usually less severe than that seen with rotavirus infection.

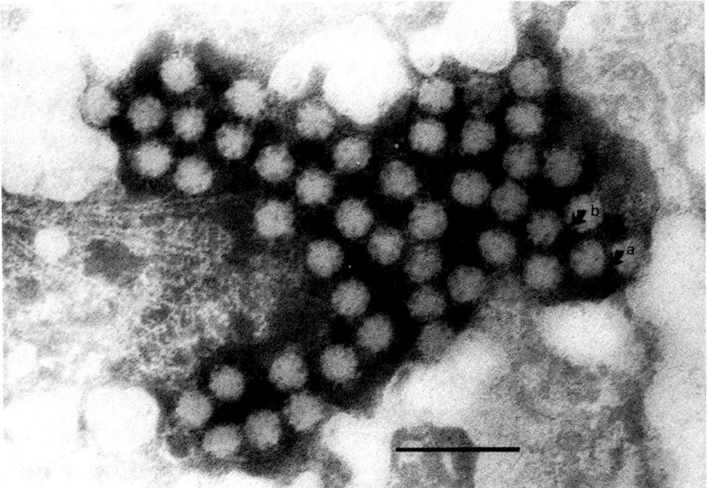

Fig. 3.80 Astrovirus. Electron micrograph showing negatively-stained particles of 28–32 nm diameter in faeces. Surface morphology shows both 5- and 6-pointed stars. Bar = 100 nm. By courtesy of Regional Virus Laboratory, East Birmingham Hospital Birmingham, England.

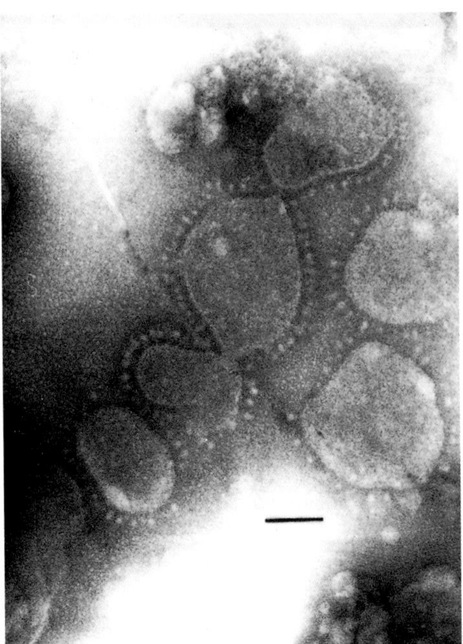

Fig. 3.81 Coronavirus. Electron micrograph showing negatively-stained pleomorphic particles which can vary in size from 80–300 nm in diameter. The particles are covered by evenly spaced pin-like projections which can look like a fringe or 'crown'. Bar = 100 nm. By courtesy of Regional Virus Laboratory, East Birmingham Hospital Birmingham, England.

Coronaviruses are enveloped, single-stranded RNA viruses approximately 80–150 nm in diameter which are well-documented causes of upper respiratory tract illness. Projections on the surface of the rounded particles give the appearance of the corona of the sun. Coronavirus-like particles have been seen by direct EM in the stools of patients with acute non-bacterial gastroenteritis (Fig. 3.81). The evidence that these agents cause acute gastroenteritis consists of the findings that in certain areas, such as southern Arizona in the USA, coronavirus-like particles are seen much more frequently in the stools of patients with diarrhoea than in healthy individuals; convalescent serum from these patients reacts with certain coronaviruses. These enteric coronavirus-like agents cannot be propagated in routine cell types and most investigators have not been able to propagate them at all. Most cases of diarrhoea associated with these agents occur in children less than 2 years old; the illness is usually dominated by diarrhoea, with or without vomiting.

CYTOMEGALOVIRUS COLITIS

Colitis due to infection with cytomegalovirus (CMV) is seen almost exclusively in patients with suppression of the immune system. At least 5–10% of patients with AIDS develop CMV colitis. In about one-third of the cases CMV colitis is the initial opportunistic infection experienced by the patient. Nearly all patients have diarrhoea and abdominal pain. Colonoscopy reveals focal or diffuse areas of erythema, mucosal oedema and mucosal erosion. Haemorrhage and mucosal ulcers 5–10 mm in diameter are commonly observed. Diagnosis of CMV colitis can be made only by biopsy of colonic or rectal mucosa. Typical findings are CMV inclusions in swollen endothelial cells associated with neutrophilic infiltration of blood vessels (Fig. 3.82). CMV can often be cultured from biopsy specimens. Isolation of CMV from stool cultures is not adequate to establish the diagnosis of CMV colitis.

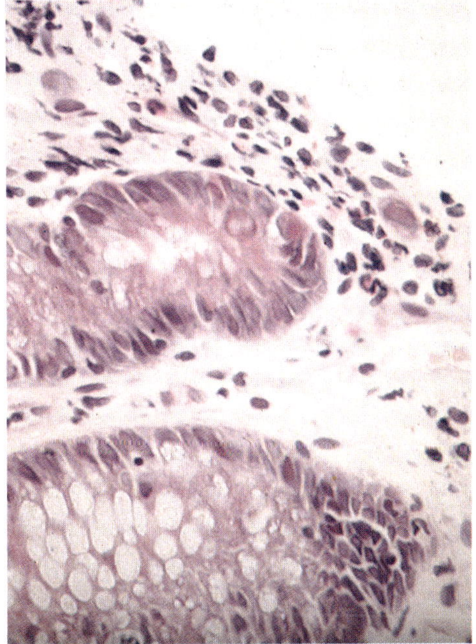

Fig. 3.82 Cytomegalovirus colitis. Section of colon showing several giant cells with eosinophilic intranuclear inclusions and infiltration of inflammatory cells in the lamina propria. By courtesy of Dr C. Edwards.

Many patients with CMV colitis associated with AIDS have now been treated with the antiviral agent ganciclovir and a majority have had a clinical response with decrease in diarrhoea and abdominal pain. Unless maintenance therapy is continued for an indefinite period, clinical and virological relapse usually occurs.

Chapter 4

Infections of the Peritoneum and Peritoneal Cavity

APPENDICITIS

Acute appendicitis is due to acute inflammation of the wall of the appendix, usually associated with some degree of obstruction of the appendiceal lumen. Classic clinical findings are tenderness at or near McBurney's point in the right lower quadrant of the abdomen, with rebound tenderness, voluntary guarding or rigidity, low-grade fever and leucocytosis. Anatomically, there is frequently an obstructing faecalith in the lumen of the appendix with distension of the lumen, infiltration with acute inflammatory cells and oedema in the wall, and hyperaemia and petechial haemorrhages on the serosal surface (Figs 4.1 & 4.2). Persistent obstruction of the appendiceal lumen by a faecalith leads eventually to gangrene and rupture of the appendix (Figs 4.3 & 4.4). Spillage of pus from the inflamed appendix into the peritoneal cavity may result in generalized peritonitis; alternatively the infection may be walled off with formation of an appendiceal abscess (Fig. 4.5).

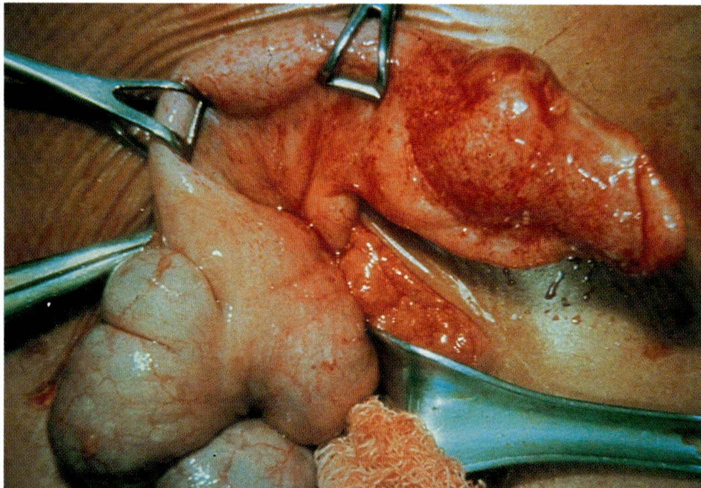

Fig. 4.1 Acute appendicitis. Operating room photograph showing a globoid tip secondary to obstruction of appendiceal lumen by a faecalith. There is pronounced hyperaemia and oedema of the appendix wall with petechial haemorrhages on the surface and dilatation of the lumen distal to the obstruction. By courtesy of Dr M. Anderson.

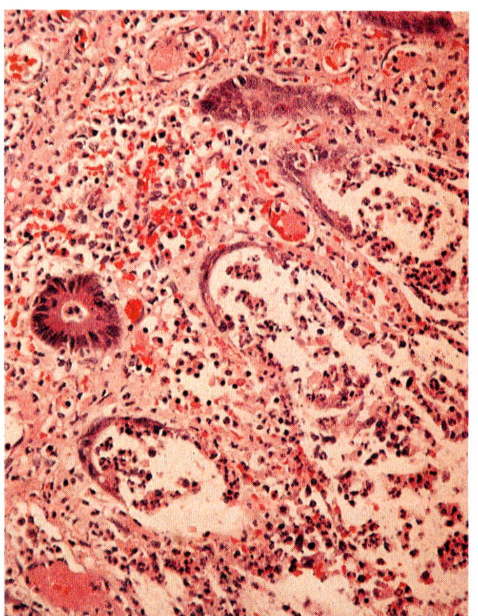

Fig. 4.2 Acute appendicitis. Histological section of the wall of the appendix showing acute inflammation, destruction of glands and intense vascular congestion with fibrin microthrombi. H&E stain.

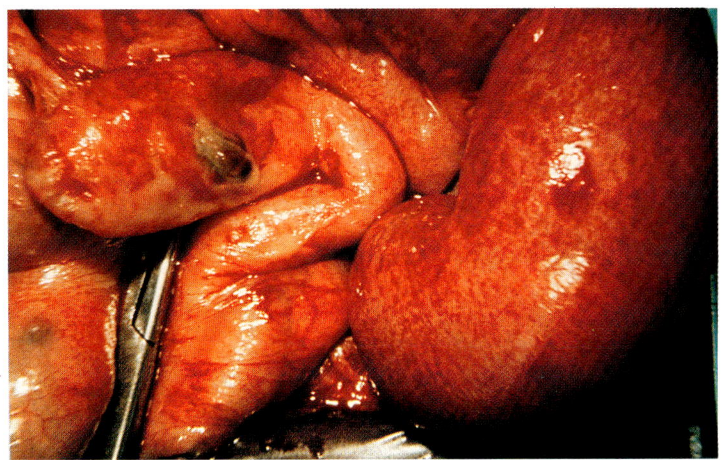

Fig. 4.3 Acute appendicitis. Operating room photograph showing an area of necrosis in the wall of the appendix with perforation at the site of obstruction by a faecalith. There is vascular congestion and fibrinous exudate on the adjacent serosal surface. By courtesy of Dr M. Anderson.

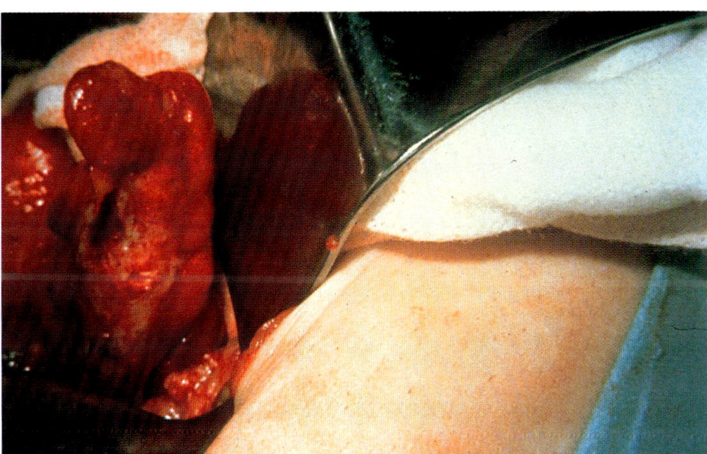

Fig. 4.4 Acute appendicitis. Operating room photograph showing acute gangrenous appendicitis with intense hyperaemia of the serosal surface of the appendix and a creamy exudate on the surface. Perforation has occurred in the middle third of the appendix, and there is a greenish gangrenous area adjacent to the perforation. By courtesy of Dr W. M. Rambo.

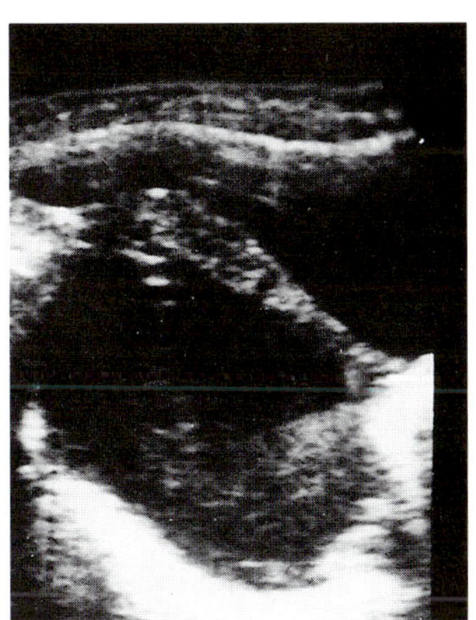
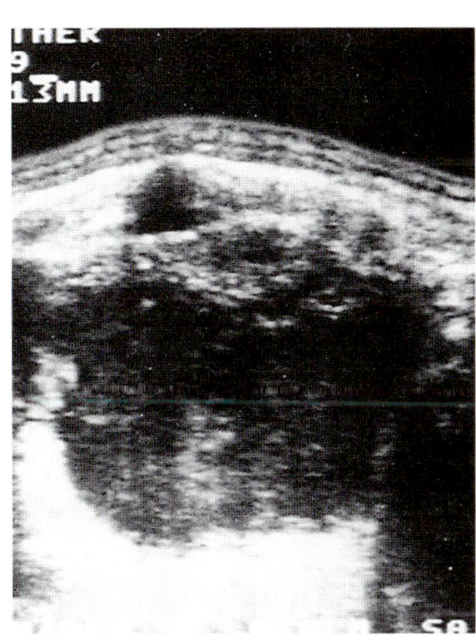

Fig. 4.5 Appendiceal abscess. Ultrasound studies showing an abscess in the pouch of Douglas secondary to a ruptured appendix. Lateral view (left) and transverse view (right). By courtesy of Dr A. E. A. Joseph.

PERITONITIS AND INTRA-ABDOMINAL ABSCESS

Primary peritonitis, in which no primary focus of infection is apparent, occurs most commonly in association with alcoholic cirrhosis and ascites. *E. coli* and related species are isolated most frequently. Spread of infection from an intra-abdominal organ into the peritoneal space results in secondary peritonitis (Fig. 4.6). Organisms may reach the peritoneal cavity either by transmural spread through the intact wall of a severely inflamed viscus, or by rupture of a viscus with spillage of its contents into the surrounding space. The intense inflammatory response of the peritoneum to bacterial infection includes deposi-tion of fibrin and migration of polymorphonuclear leucocytes, both of which tend to limit the spread of bacteria to a localized area. Complete walling off of the infection without eradication of the microorganisms results in formation of an intra-abdominal abscess. In addition to appendicitis, important sources for peritonitis and intra-abdominal abscess include rupture of the gallbladder, perforation of a peptic ulcer, ruptured intestinal diverticulum, acute pancreatitis, chronic peritoneal dialysis (Fig. 4.7) and pelvic inflammatory disease. Most cases of secondary peritonitis are polymicrobial, with mixtures of anaerobic and facultative enteric bacteria. New imaging methods such as CT scanning (Fig. 4.8), radionuclide scanning (Figs 4.9 & 4.10) and

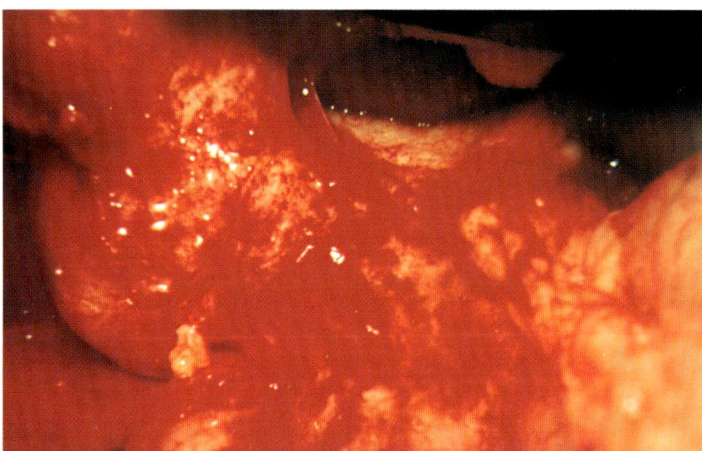

Fig. 4.6 Acute peritonitis. Operating room photograph showing localized acute peritoneal inflammation with oedema, acute inflammatory exudate, intense vascular congestion and petechial haemorrhage, associated with acute cholecystitis. By courtesy of Dr M. Anderson.

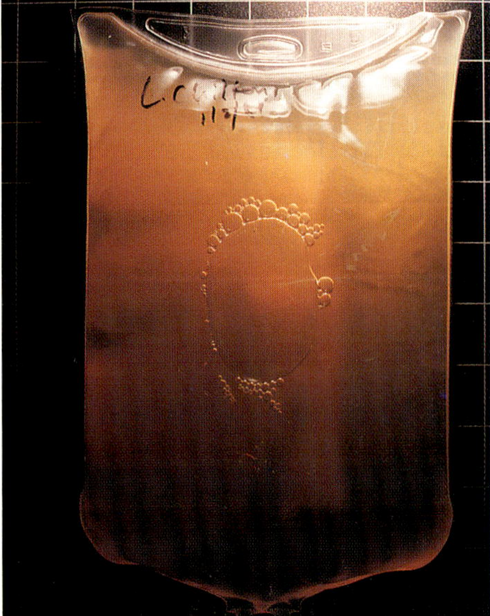

Fig. 4.7 Acute peritonitis. Cloudy, infected peritoneal dialysate removed from a patient undergoing chronic peritoneal dialysis.

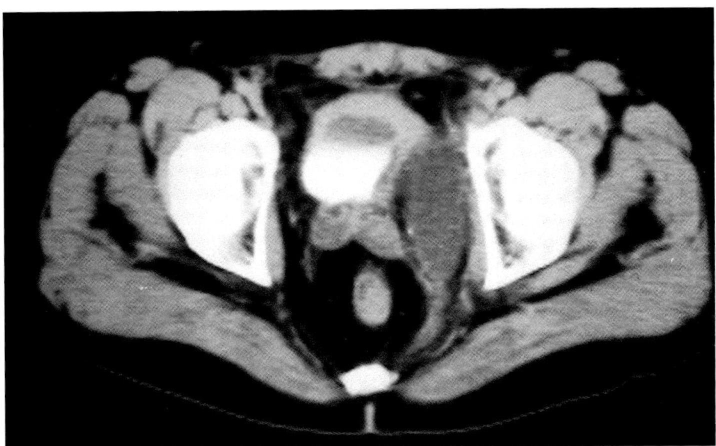

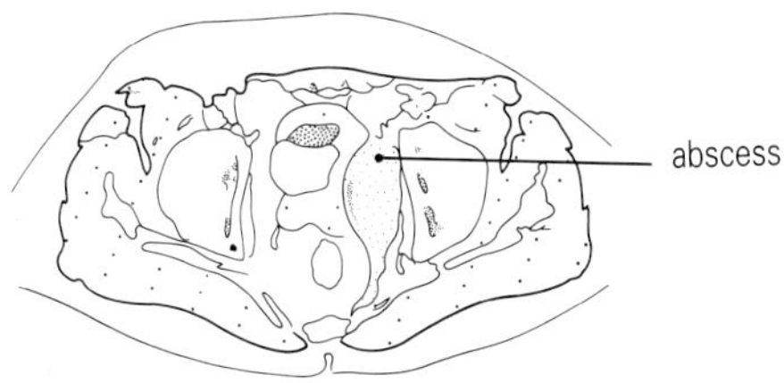

Fig. 4.8 Intra-abdominal abscess. CT scan at the level of the seminal vesicles showing an elliptical abscess to the left of the midline.

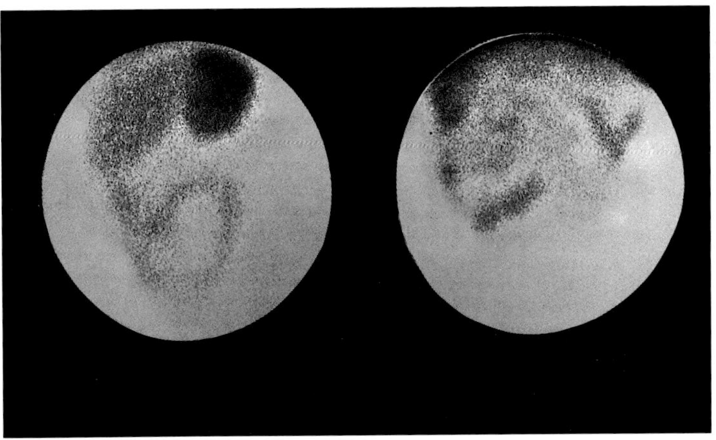

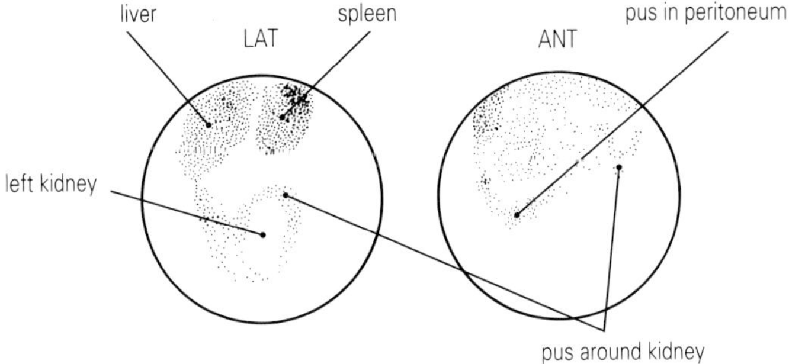

Fig. 4.9 Intra-abdominal abscess. Leucocytes labelled with indium-111 have concentrated in regions of purulent peritoneal fluid. Activity is normally seen by this technique in the liver and spleen. By courtesy of Dr D. Ackery.

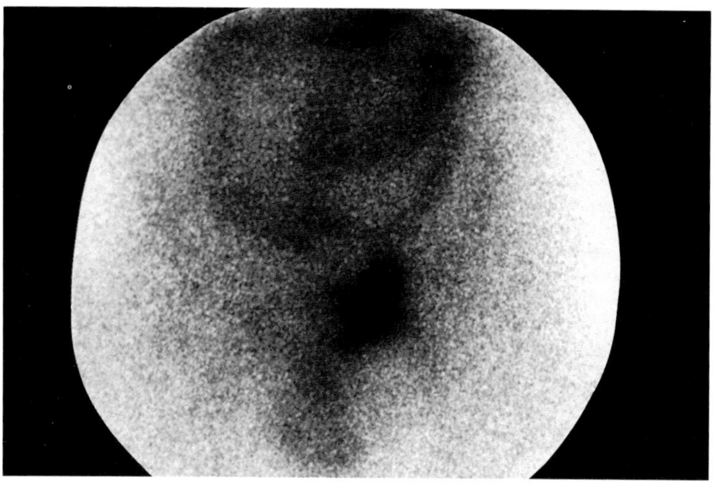

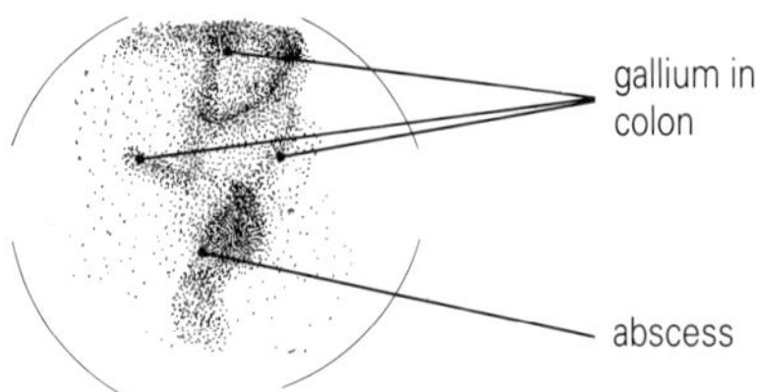

Fig. 4.10 Intra-abdominal abscess. Gallium scan showing an area of increased uptake of the radionuclide in the left lower quadrant of the abdomen. Gallium is also seen in the lumen of the colon.

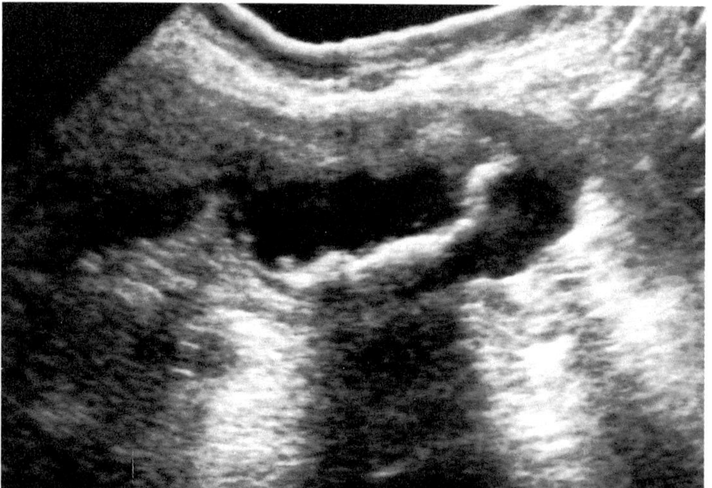

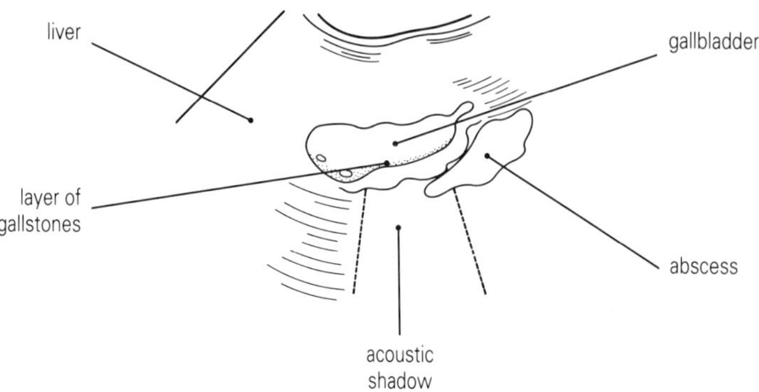

Fig. 4.11 Pericholecystic abscess. Ultrasound study showing sonolucent abscess cavity adjacent to the gallbladder in a patient with a pericholecystic abscess secondary to perforation of the gallbladder. By courtesy of Dr A. E. A. Joseph.

ultrasound studies (Fig. 4.11) have greatly facilitated the prompt and accurate diagnosis of intra-abdominal abscess. Empirical treatment of secondary peritonitis should include an agent or agents active against both anaerobic and facultative organisms, such as imipenem or a combination of metronidazole or clindamycin with a third-generation cephalosporin. If abscess formation has occurred, catheter or surgical drainage will also be required.

Tuberculous peritonitis

Tuberculous peritonitis is usually due to rupture of a caseous abdominal lymph node. It may or may not be accompanied by active pulmonary disease. Pleural effusion is frequently present. The peritoneal disease may be manifested by abdominal masses and a doughy abdomen or by presence of ascites and signs of peritonitis. Low-grade fever, anorexia, weight loss and abdominal pain are common. The clinical picture may mimic many other intra-abdominal diseases, and the diagnosis is particularly difficult in the presence of co-existing cirrhosis with ascites and in patients undergoing chronic peritoneal dialysis. The tuberculin test is often negative. The peritoneal fluid usually contains 500–2000 cells, predominantly lymphocytes. Smears of the fluid are rarely positive and culture yields *M. tuberculosis* in only 25% of cases. Surgical exploration or laparoscopy often reveals fibrous adhesions, ascites and tubercles scattered over the peritoneal surface (Figs 4.12, 4.13 & 4.14) and biopsy of these lesions yields the diagnosis in up to 85% of cases. Treatment is the same as for pulmonary tuberculosis.

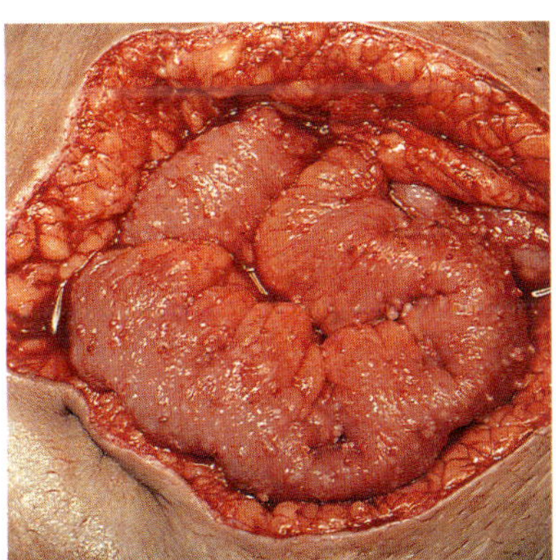

Fig. 4.12 Tuberculous peritonitis. Operating room photograph showing oedematous bowel with numerous focal white lesions on the peritoneal surface. By courtesy of Dr M. Goldman.

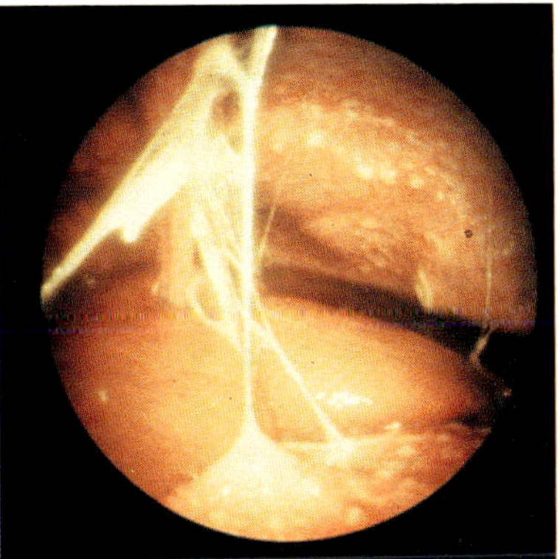

Fig. 4.13 Tuberculous peritonitis. Laparoscopic view in a patient with the chronic serous type of TB peritonitis, showing fibrous adhesions attached to the left lobe of the liver and numerous tubercles on the parietal peritoneum. By courtesy of Dr J. Cunningham.

ABDOMINAL ACTINOMYCOSIS

Abdominal actinomycosis usually occurs following abdominal surgery, trauma or rupture of a colonic diverticulum or duodenal ulcer. The latent period between this event and subsequent development of manifestations of actinomycosis may be several years, so the connection between the two is not always immediately apparent. The ileocaecal region is most frequently involved and the lesion may be

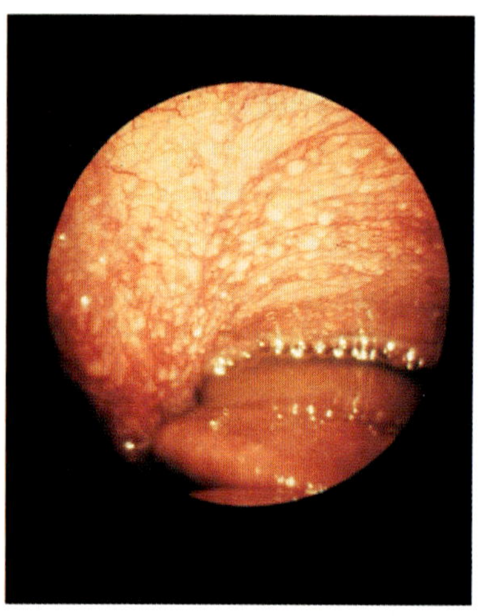

Fig. 4.14 Tuberculous peritonitis. Laparoscopic view in a patient with extensive acute exudative tuberculous peritonitis, showing vascular engorgement, multiple granulomas on the parietal peritoneum and ascites. By courtesy of Dr J. Cunningham.

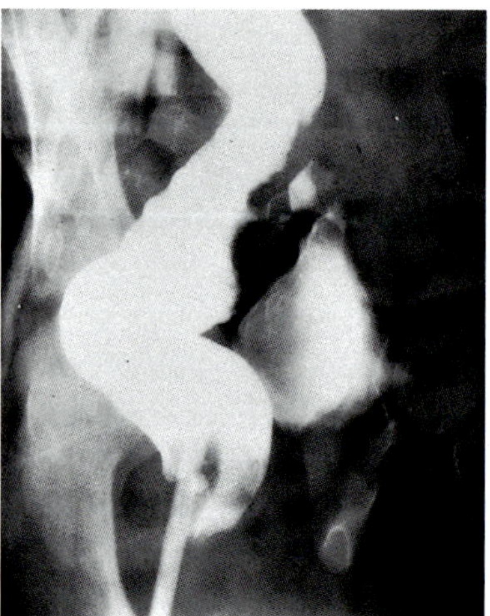

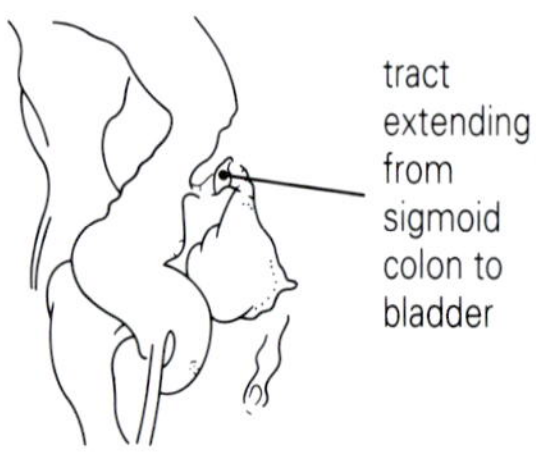

Fig. 4.15 Abdominal actinomycosis. Barium enema showing an area of mucosal abnormality in the sigmoid colon, with a fistulous tract extending from the sigmoid colon to the urinary bladder, which is filled with contrast material.

mistaken for a caecal carcinoma, tuberculosis or amoebiasis. A mass lesion is frequently produced with contiguous spread and fistula formation involving the body wall, perianal region or other internal organs (Fig. 4.15). Pus obtained by aspiration or surgical drainage may reveal sulphur granules (Fig. 4.16). Gram's stain reveals the characteristic beaded, filamentous, gram-positive organisms (Fig. 4.17) and *Actinomyces israelii* can be grown anaerobically.

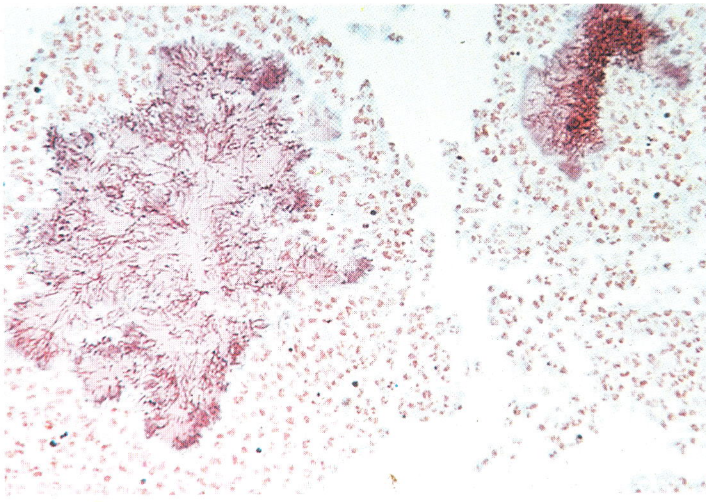

Fig. 4.16 Abdominal actinomycosis. Inflammatory exudate containing a typical sulphur granule. By courtesy of Dr C. Edwards.

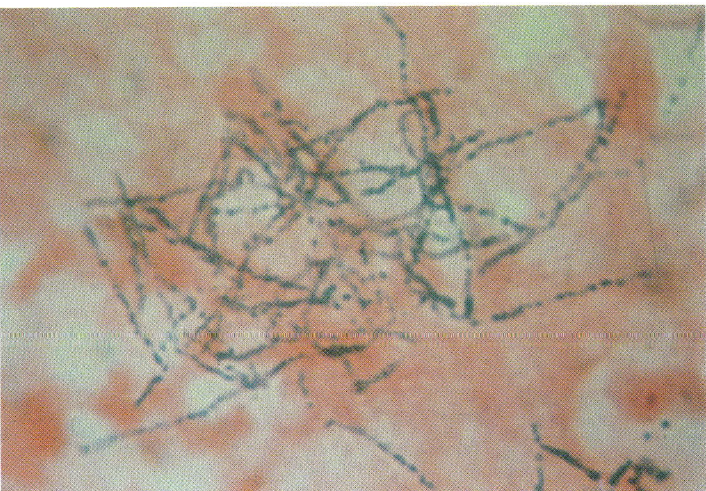

Fig. 4.17 Abdominal actinomycosis. Pus drained from an intra-abdominal abscess showing tangled, beaded, gram-positive filaments of *Actinomyces israelii*. Gram's stain. By courtesy of A. E. Prevost.

ECHINOCOCCOSIS

Echinococcosis (hydatid disease) is caused by human infection with the tapeworm *Echinococcus granulosus.* Man becomes involved accidentally by ingesting the eggs which are present in the faeces of infected dogs. The most common location of hydatid cysts is the liver, usually the right lobe, followed by the lung. Usually a single cyst is present.

Rupture of the cyst through the capsule of the liver into the peritoneal cavity results in the formation of new daughter cysts throughout the peritoneum and omentum (Fig. 4.18). Rupture through the diaphragm may lead to dissemination throughout the pleural space. The new larvae (scolices – Fig. 4.19) develop in large numbers from the germinal layer of brood capsules within the wall of the cyst.

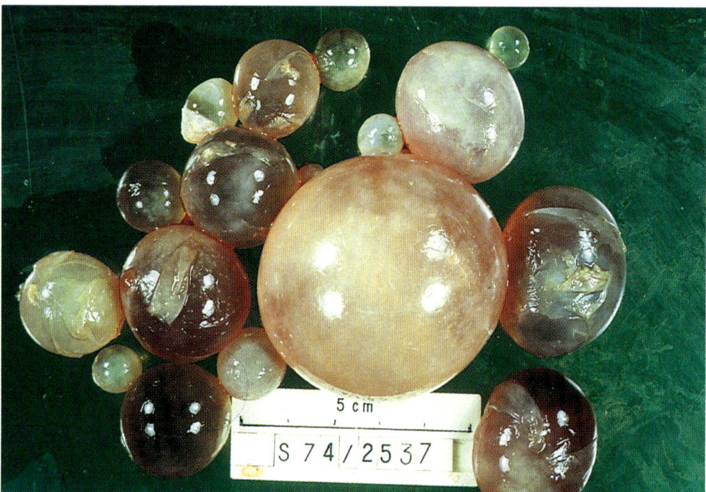

Fig. 4.18 Echinococcosis. Surgical specimen showing multiple hydatid cysts from the omentum of a patient who had infection disseminated throughout the peritoneal cavity.

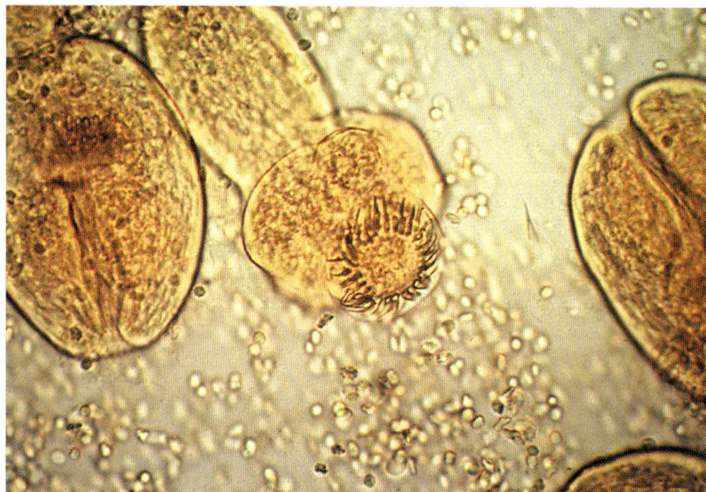

Fig. 4.19 Echinococcosis. Light microscopy of scolices from a hydatid cyst showing both invaginated and evaginated hooklets and suckers. By courtesy of Prof. W. Peters.

Chapter 5

Infections of the Liver

ACUTE HEPATITIS

Acute hepatitis may be caused by a large number of different viruses, the most important of which are the hepatitis B virus (HBV), the hepatitis A virus (HAV) and the non-A, non-B (NANB) group. Clinical and morphological features of all three types of infection are similar. Hepatitis is the pre-

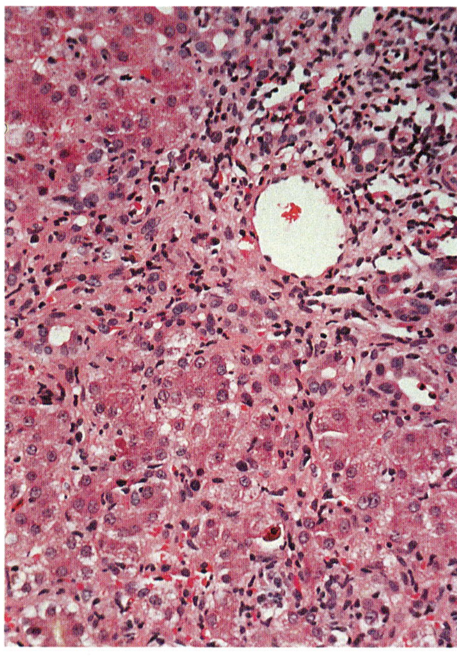

Fig. 5.1 Acute viral hepatitis. Histological section of liver showing hepatocytes in degeneration, necrosis and regeneration. H&E stain. By courtesy of Dr R. D. Johnson.

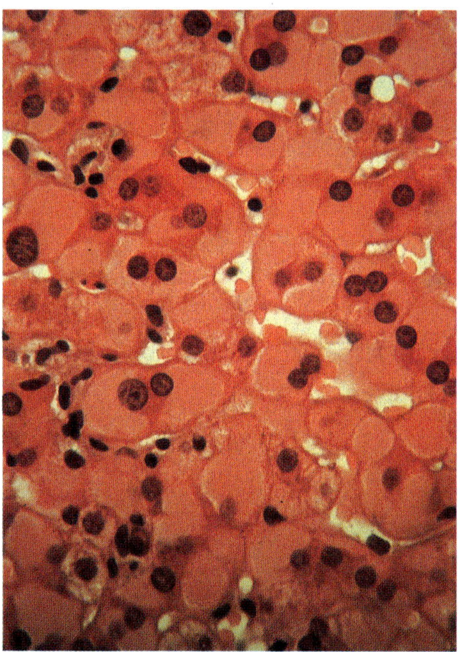

Fig. 5.2 Viral hepatitis. Histological section of liver showing 'ground-glass' hepatocytes. H&E stain.

dominant manifestation of yellow fever, and is a common feature of cytomegalovirus infection and infectious mononucleosis, caused by the Epstein–Barr virus. Less commonly, the liver may be involved in disseminated herpes simplex infection and in varicella (chickenpox). Nonviral forms of acute hepatitis include Q fever, bacterial hepatitis, leptospirosis and Reye's syndrome.

Pathologically, viral hepatitis is characterized by spotty necrosis scattered throughout the liver lobule with varying degrees of degeneration of liver cells, including necrosis, infiltration of the liver by mononuclear cells and variable degrees of cholestasis (Fig. 5.1). In HBV infections, 'ground-glass' hepatocytes and specific staining of HBV surface antigen may be demonstrated (Figs 5.2 & 5.3). Hepatic cell necrosis is usually focal and limited in extent, but occasionally, especially in HBV infection, massive hepatic necrosis (acute yellow atrophy) occurs with loss of nearly all liver cells and complete collapse of the hepatic architecture (Figs 5.4 and 5.5). As discussed below, some types of viral hepatitis may persist and produce chronic lesions in the liver, including postnecrotic cirrhosis.

Hepatitis B Virus

Infection with HBV (hepatitis B), formerly known as serum hepatitis, is the most prevalent type of acute hepatitis worldwide. Persistent infection with the virus is common, and in highly endemic areas approximately 10% of the population are chronic carriers of HBV; in many individuals infection persists for life. The total number of chronic carriers worldwide exceeds 230 million. Formerly a major cause of transfusion-associated hepatitis, HBV infection is now most frequently spread by sexual contact, intravenous drug abuse and transmission from mothers to their newborn infants.

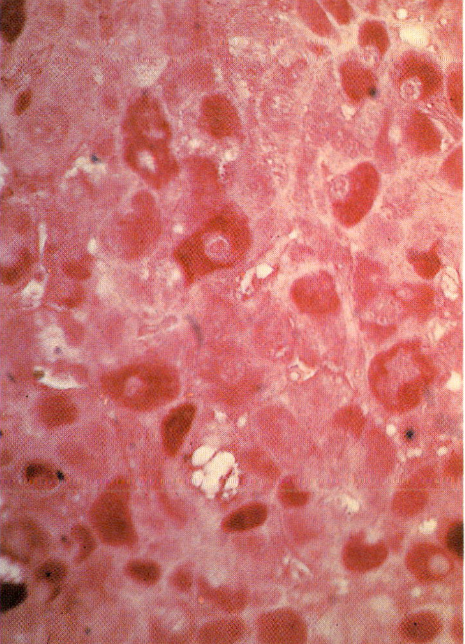

Fig. 5.3 Viral hepatitis. Histological section of liver in hepatitis B virus infection showing specific staining of hepatitis B surface antigen in hepatocytes. Shikata stain. By courtesy of Dr R. D. Johnson.

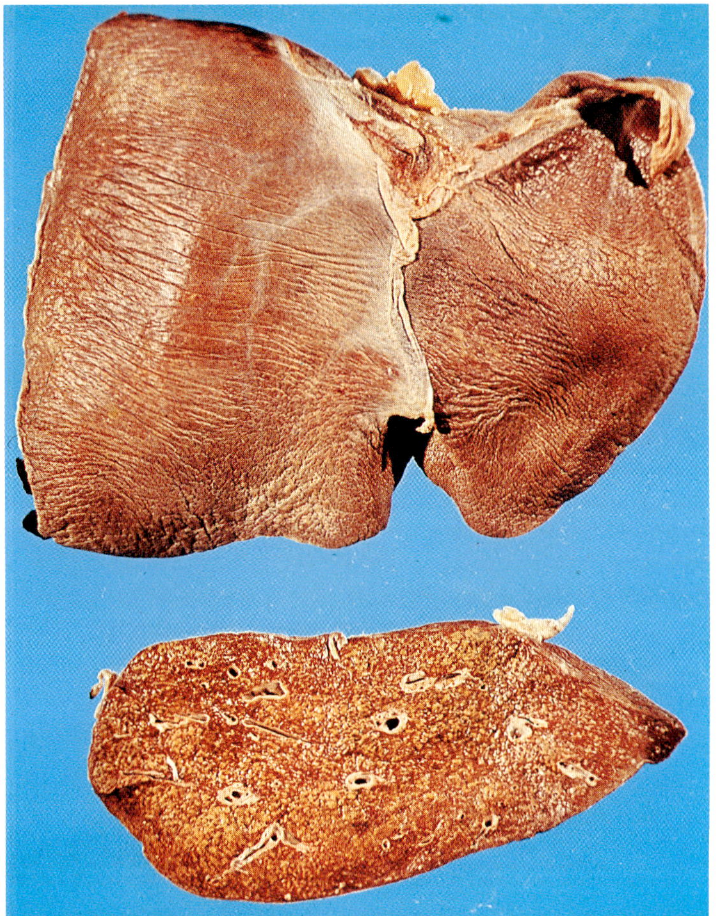

Fig. 5.4 Viral hepatitis. Gross specimen of liver showing massive hepatic necrosis. The capsular surface (upper) is wrinkled. The cut surface (lower) has a 'nutmeg' appearance due to cell loss and congestion in the central lobular zones. Light foci represent remaining liver cells; areas of necrosis appear darker. The hepatic architecture has collapsed and the organ has shrunk in size. By courtesy of Dr J. Newman.

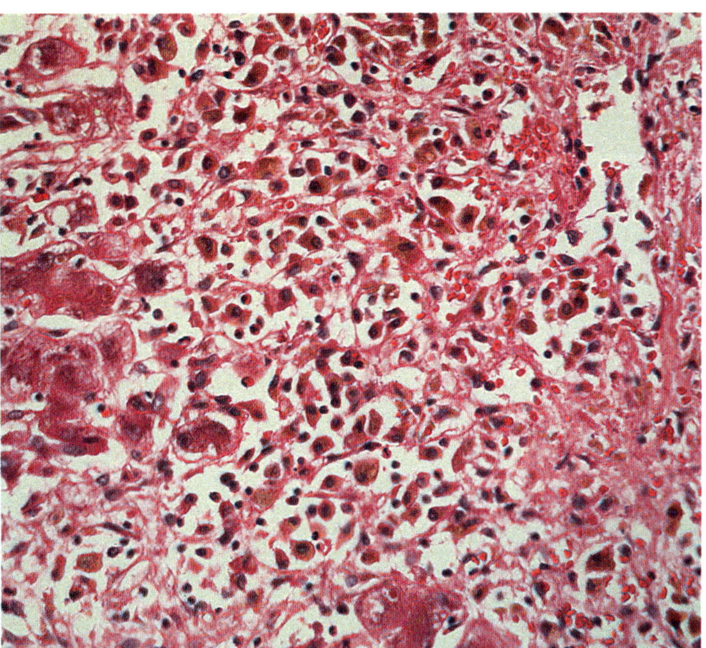

Fig. 5.5 Viral hepatitis. Histological section of liver showing massive hepatic necrosis due to hepatitis A virus infection. There is a paucity of hepatocytes and large numbers of pigment-laden macrophages. H&E stain. By courtesy of Dr R. D. Johnson.

Three types of viral particles are found in the blood of infected individuals (Fig. 5.6). The complete virion (Dane particle) is 42 nm in diameter. The hepatitis B surface antigen particle (HB$_s$Ag), which may be spherical, filamentous or rod-shaped, is 22 nm in diameter. The virion core, also 22 nm in diameter, contains the core antigen (HB$_c$Ag), the viral DNA, DNA polymerase, protein kinase activity and the 'e' antigen (HB$_e$Ag), which is closely associated with infectivity. The genome of HBV is complex and unique; its replication involves the activity of reverse transcriptase which is unique among human DNA viruses. This replication mechanism, and the nucleotide sequence homology between HBV and retroviruses, suggests a possible phylogenetic relationship between these two families of viruses.

Man is the only important reservoir of HBV. Blood and blood products are the best documented sources of the virus, but it is also found in faeces, urine, bile, semen, saliva and other body fluids. The most important vehicles for infection are probably blood, semen and saliva. Transmission commonly occurs via percutaneous inoculation of virus during administration of contaminated blood or blood products, haemodialysis, tattooing, ear piercing, acupuncture, sharing of needles by intravenous drug abusers, or accidental needle stick injuries by hospital personnel, and also during heterosexual and homosexual contact. In areas of the world where the prevalence of chronic HBV infection is very high, transmission from infected mothers to infants occurs frequently during late pregnancy, parturition or during the first two months' postpartum.

The incubation period of acute hepatitis B is usually between 2–6 months. In patients who develop jaundice, 10–20% have a prodromal serum-sickness-like illness with fever, maculopapular erythematous rash, arthralgias and urticaria for several days to several weeks before the appearance of signs of liver disease.

The severity of acute hepatitis B varies widely, and many cases are clinically inapparent. In these subclinical cases and in anicteric cases, serum transaminases are usually elevated. In icteric cases malaise, fever, headache, anorexia and nausea, sometimes with vomiting, appear 2–7 days before the appearance of jaundice. Anorexia is often pronounced and accompanied by an aversion for tobacco; the smell of food or tobacco may induce nausea. Pain and tenderness in the right upper quadrant are common. The liver is often enlarged, palpable and tender. Icterus of the sclerae and other mucous membranes and skin are usually noted when the concentration of serum bilirubin is ⩾3 mg/100 ml.

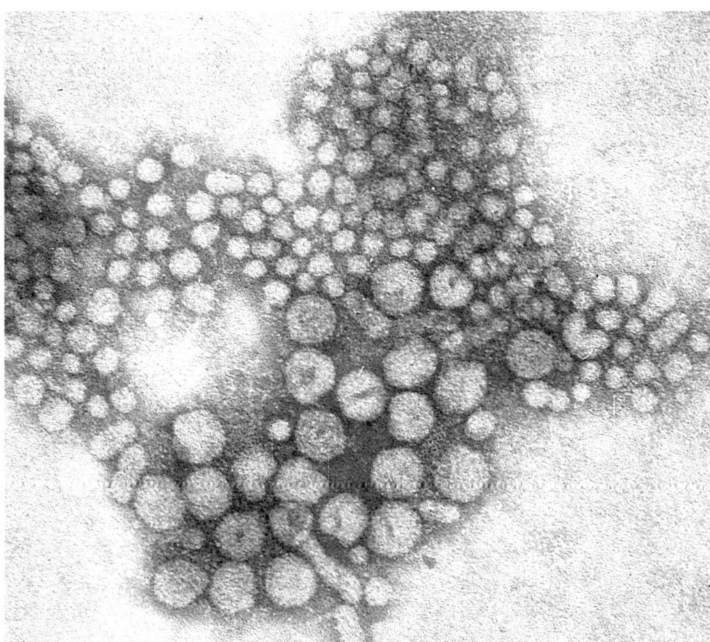

Fig. 5.6 Viral hepatitis. Electron micrograph of hepatitis B virus, serum specimen. The smaller rounded structures are non-infectious particles containing HB$_s$Ag determinant on their surfaces. HB$_s$Ag can also be seen in tubular or filamentous form. The larger (40–50 nm diameter) rounded bodies are Dane particles, probably the fully assembled infectious virus. By courtesy of Professor C. R. Madely.

Laboratory abnormalities include a striking increase in serum transaminases (SGPT > SGOT), with a peak of 1000 U/ml or greater reached within the first week of illness. Serum bilirubin rises during the first 10–14 days and then declines over the next 2–4 weeks in most cases.

Although most cases of hepatitis B have a relatively mild and self-limited course, fulminant hepatitis with hepatic failure and encephalopathy may occur. The case fatality rate is very high, with death usually occurring within three weeks of onset. Infection with a variant HBV containing a stop-

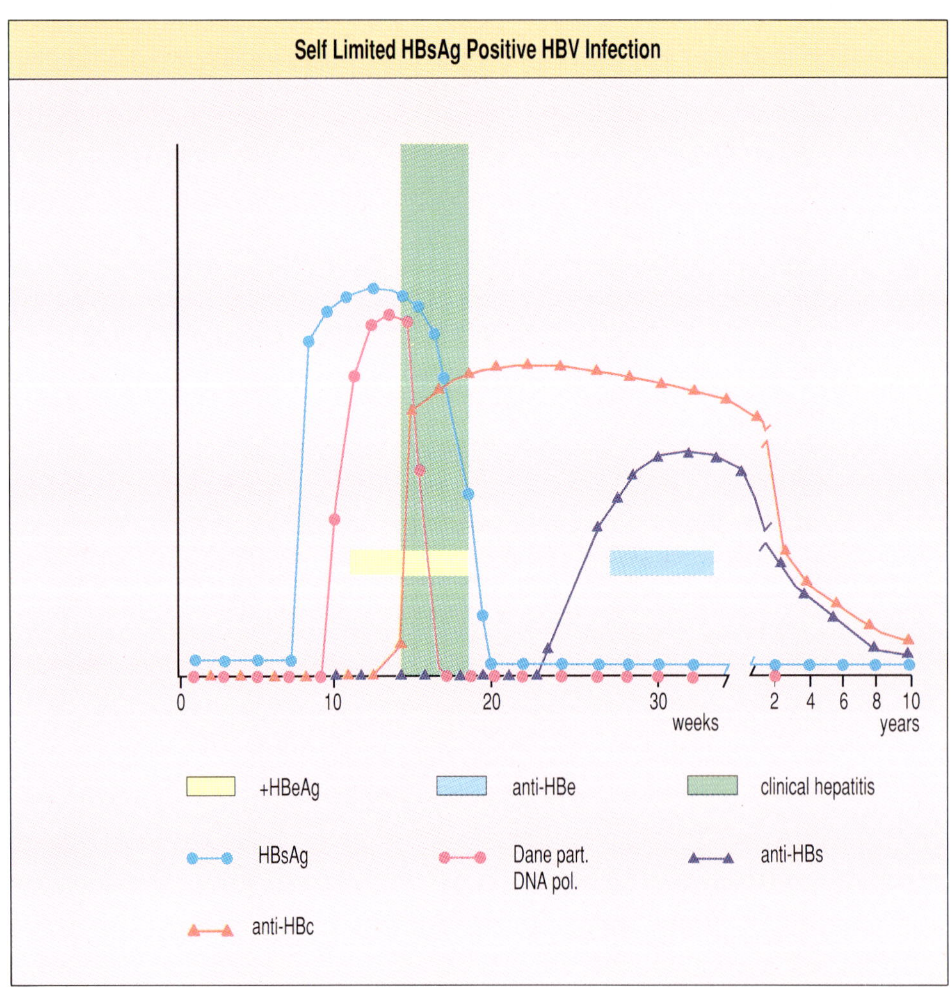

Fig. 5.7 Hepatitis B. Schematic representation of viral markers in the blood throughout the course of self-limited, HB$_s$Ag-positive primary HBV infection. Adapted from Robinson WS. Hepatitis B virus and hepatitis delta virus. In: Mandell GL, Douglas RG, Bennett JE, eds. *Principles and Practice of Infectious Diseases, Third Edition*, Churchill Livingstone, New York, 1990.

codon mutation involving the pre-core region of the viral genome or concomitant infection with hepatitis delta virus (HDV) (see below) is associated with an increased risk of fulminant hepatitis.

During the active stage of self-limited hepatitis, both HB$_s$Ag and HB$_e$Ag can be detected in the blood. These antigens disappear after weeks or months, and antibodies against surface antigen (anti-HB$_s$), core antigen (anti-HB$_c$) and 'e' antigen (anti-HB$_e$) appear and persist, at gradually declining titres, for years (Fig. 5.7). In persistent infection HB$_s$Ag, with or without HB$_e$Ag, persists indefinitely. Anti-HB$_c$ and anti-HB$_e$ are also present, but not anti-HB$_s$ (Fig. 5.8).

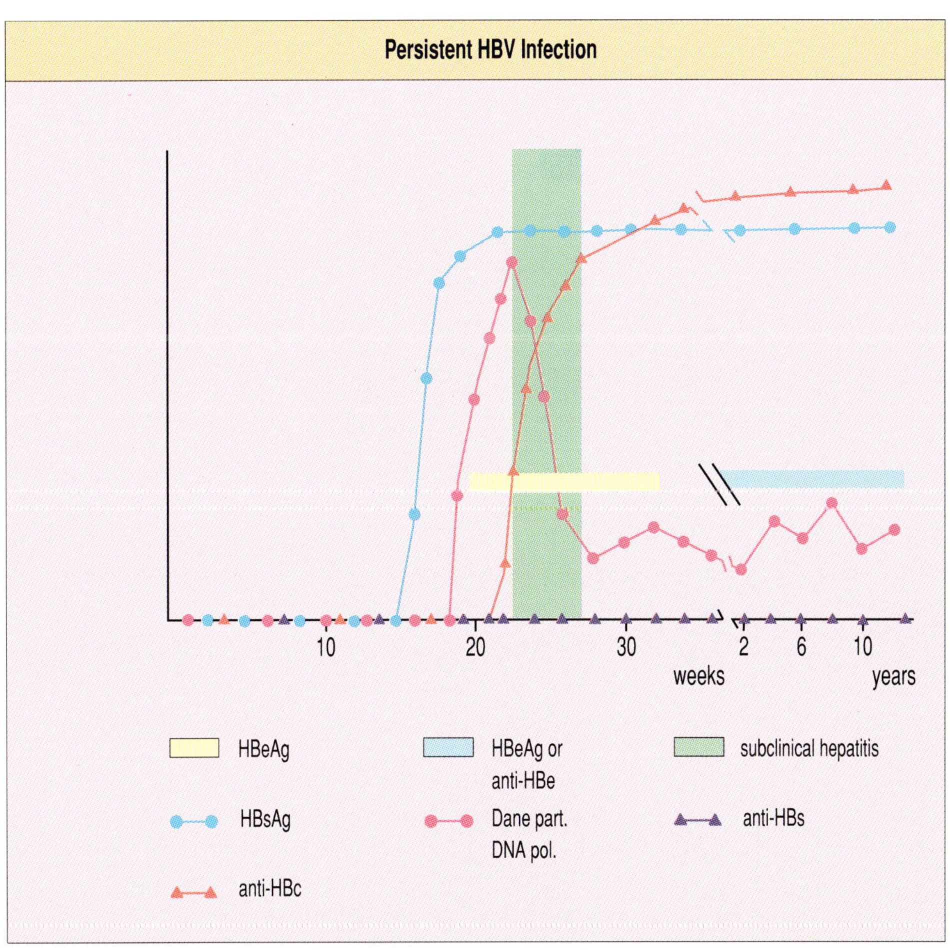

Fig. 5.8 Hepatitis B. Schematic representation of viral markers in the blood throughout the course of HBV infection that becomes persistent. For source see Fig. 5.7.

In 5–10% of adults, and virtually 100% of new-borns, persistent infection occurs. This may be associated with a histologically normal liver and normal liver function, but it often results in lesions designated 'chronic persistent' hepatitis, in which the basic hepatic architecture is preserved (Fig. 5.9), or 'chronic active' hepatitis in which there is disruption of lobular architecture and degeneration and regeneration of hepatocytes (Fig. 5.10). The presence of HB_eAg in persistent infection is usually associated with chronic hepatitis. Chronic active hepatitis may eventually result in postnecrotic cirrhosis, with extensive fibrosis and distortion of the lobular architecture of the liver.

Hepatitis B infection is also closely associated with development of hepatocellular carcinoma which, after skin cancer, is the most common malignant tumour worldwide. Hepatitis B viral DNA, often integrated into the genome of liver cells, can be demonstrated in approximately 75% of hepatocellular carcinoma cases; exactly how the virus is involved in carcinogenesis is not known. Extrahepatic manifestations of persistent HBV infection, possibly related to circulating immune complexes, include a serum sickness-like syndrome, polyarteritis nodosa and membranous glomerulonephritis.

Vaccines prepared from heat-inactivated serum containing HB_sAg, or by recombinant DNA techniques, provide effective protection against HBV infection. Immunization is of no value in individuals with pre-existing antibody to HB_sAg or in chronic

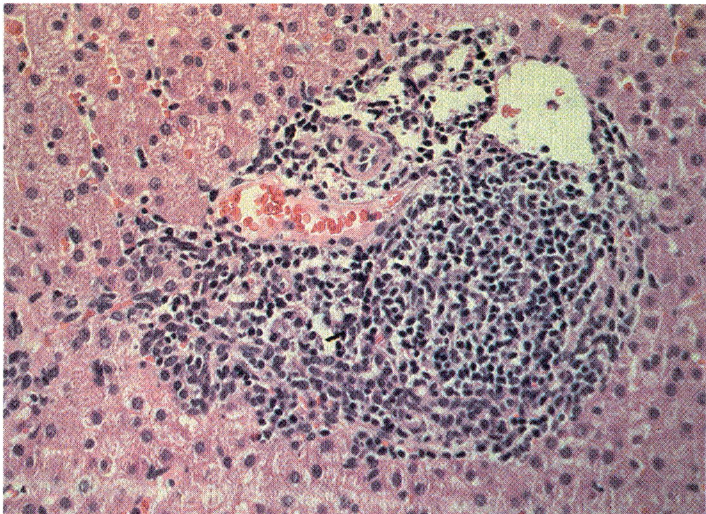

Fig. 5.9 Chronic persistent hepatitis. Histological section of liver showing inflammatory nodule in a portal triad. Hepatic architecture is otherwise preserved and the limiting plate is intact. H&E stain. By courtesy of Dr R. D. Johnson.

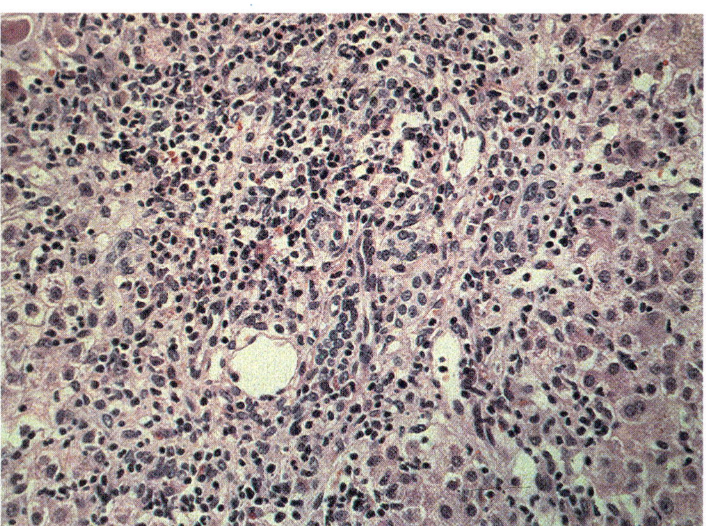

Fig. 5.10 Chronic active hepatitis. Histological section of liver showing extensive infiltration by inflammatory cells with loss of the limiting plate, disruption of lobular architecture and degeneration and regeneration of hepatocytes. H&E stain. By courtesy of Dr R. D. Johnson.

HB$_s$Ag carriers. Administration of hepatitis B vaccine is recommended particularly for individuals with a high risk of infection, such as male homosexuals, intravenous drug abusers, household and sexual contacts of hepatitis B carriers, dialysis patients, recipients of clotting factors VIII or IX, medical and laboratory workers with frequent exposure to blood or blood products, mortuary workers, and residents and staff members of institutions for the mentally retarded. Adults should receive 1 ml vaccine intramuscularly at 0, 1 and 6 months; children under 10 years should receive 0.5 ml on the same schedule. If exposure to HBV occurs via needle stick injury, or by other means such as sexual intercourse, oral exchange of saliva by kissing or sharing a toothbrush of an unimmunized individual, prompt administration of serum immune globulin with high titres of anti-HB$_s$ antibody (HBIG) can provide partial protection. As soon as possible after exposure, 0.06 ml/kg HBIG should be given intramuscularly, followed either by immediate institution of active immunization with hepatitis B vaccine, or by a second dose of HBIG after 1 month.

No therapeutic measure has been shown to be beneficial in the treatment of acute viral hepatitis. Progression of chronic active hepatitis has been favourably affected by administration of corticosteroids or azathioprine. In some patients, liver function returns towards normal and cirrhosis appears to be prevented. The best results have been observed in HB$_s$Ag-negative patients, and in women treated at an early stage of disease. Unfortunately, corticosteroid therapy enhances replication of HBV, and may be associated with the appearance or rise in titre of HB$_s$Ag, HB$_e$Ag and Dane particles. Corticosteroid therapy is therefore recommended only for patients who are symptomatic, HB$_s$Ag negative and have severe histological lesions in liver biopsies.

Two antiviral agents, human leucocyte interferon-α (IFN$_\alpha$) and adenine arabinoside, have also produced beneficial results in limited trials. Further studies are required to determine their place, if any, in the treatment of chronic hepatitis B infection. Serial determination of α-fetoprotein levels and ultrasound examination of the liver in HB$_s$Ag carriers with cirrhosis may allow detection of hepatocellular carcinoma at a stage when the tumour can be cured by surgical resection.

Hepatitis A Virus

Infection with HAV, formerly known as infectious hepatitis, also occurs worldwide. The causative agent of hepatitis A is a small single-stranded RNA virus, similar to the enteroviruses, 27 nm in diameter (Fig. 5.11). Viral particles are present in hepatocytes and in faeces during the late incubation

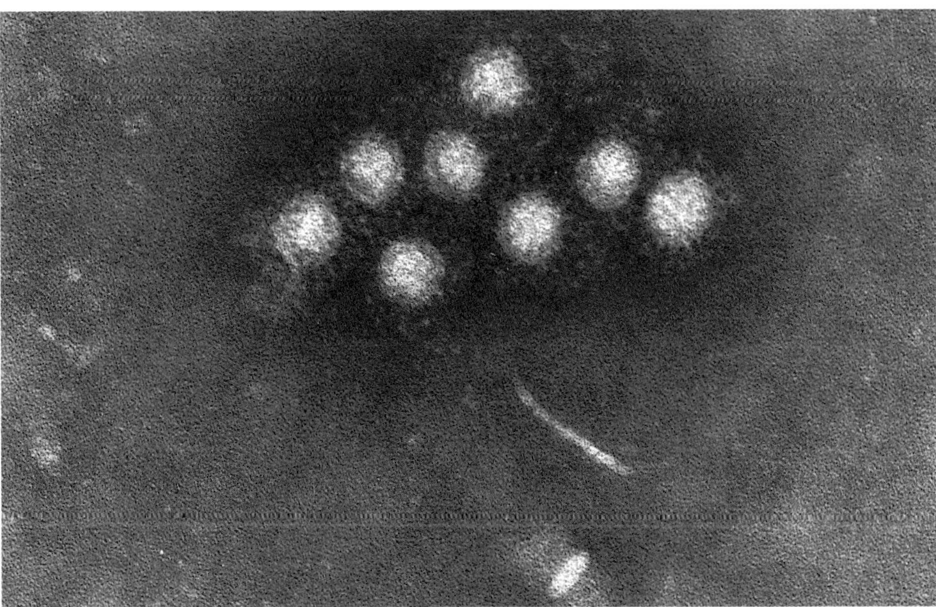

Fig. 5.11 Hepatitis A virus. Electron micrograph of negatively stained particles. Small round particles of 27 nm diameter from human faeces, agglutinated with anti-MS-1 antiserum. By courtesy of Regional Virus Laboratory, East Birmingham Hospital.

period and early stage of clinical hepatitis. Unlike HBV, with HAV there is no persistent state of infection with prolonged viraemia, so transmission by blood or blood products via parenteral routes almost never occurs. Humans represent the only significant reservoir of infection. Faeces appear to be the only important source of virus and transmission occurs most often via the faecal–oral route, or via food or water contaminated by sewage. Shellfish such as clams, oysters and mussels concentrate the virus during filter feeding and are common sources of hepatitis A infection. High risk groups include male homosexuals, children and staff members in day care centres, and other populations living in crowded settings such as prisons, military facilities and certain schools. Infection in young children is usually asymptomatic; most recognized cases occur in household contacts of children. There is little evidence for sexual transmission between heterosexual partners. The highest attack rates are found in developing countries, where housing and sanitation are inadequate. In some developing countries more than 90% of young adults have serological evidence of prior infection, as compared with approximately 20% of adults in the USA. About one-half of acute viral hepatitis cases occurring in the USA are due to HAV.

The pattern of secondary infections in household contacts of patients with hepatitis A indicates that the patient is most infectious late in the incubation period or soon after the onset of symptoms, and this corresponds with the presence of the largest numbers of viral particles in the faeces. Faecal excretion of virus ends at about the time serum transaminases rise and jaundice appears in icteric cases. Although a transient viraemia may occur late in the incubation period, percutaneous transmission by blood or serum occurs very infrequently and is insignificant as a mode of HAV transmission.

Approximately 90% of cases of HAV infection are asymptomatic. In patients who become ill the clinical picture of the acute hepatitis is indistinguishable from that produced by HBV or by NANB viruses. The incubation period is usually from 2–6 weeks. Illness begins with fever, malaise, fatigue, headache, anorexia, nausea and vomiting, myalgias and epigastric or right upper quadrant pain. Diarrhoea, arthralgias, rash and respiratory symptoms of cough, coryza, and sore throat occur occasionally. Onset of symptoms may be more abrupt in hepatitis A than in hepatitis B, in which the illness usually develops gradually. As in hepatitis B,

increased serum transaminases, dark urine and rising serum bilirubin precede the appearance of clinical jaundice. The illness usually lasts an average of two weeks, but in adults jaundice may last for one month or more. The histopathological findings are indistinguishable from those seen in acute hepatitis B. In contrast to hepatitis B, hepatitis A virus infection is not followed by chronic hepatitis.

Infection with HAV is followed by long-lasting immunity to reinfection. Serum IgG antibodies to HAV (anti-HAV) appear during the convalescent stage and persist for years; IgM antibody is present during acute infection and disappears after 3–6 months. The best method of making a serological diagnosis of hepatitis A is by detection of anti-HAV IgM antibody during or shortly after the clinical illness; IgM antibody is not likely to be acquired passively via blood transfusion.

Careful attention to hand washing and proper disposal of infectious faeces and disposal or disinfection of contaminated objects can reduce the transmission of HAV infection. Household bleach diluted 1:32 can be used to disinfect objects or surfaces contaminated with HAV. Water can be rendered non-infectious by boiling for one minute or by adequate chlorination; the concentration of chlorine required depends upon the amount of organic matter in the water. Immune globulin can provide effective pre- or post-exposure passive protection against hepatitis A infection; it is recommended for household or sexual contacts, staff of day care centres, residents and staff of prisons or institutions for the mentally retarded, and for travellers to highly endemic areas. A single injection of immune globulin, 0.02 ml/kg given intramuscularly within a few days of exposure to HAV, reduces the attack rate of clinical hepatitis A by 80–90%; protection against further exposures lasts 2–6 months. For travellers, or residents in highly endemic settings, 0.06 ml/kg given intramuscularly provides protection for at least 5 months. The dose can be repeated every 5 months. A killed virus vaccine has been developed and appears to be immunogenic, but it is not yet available for general use.

Non-A, non-B hepatitis virus

Occurrence of cases of post-transfusion hepatitis without serological evidence of either hepatitis B or A infection led to the recognition of 'non-A, non-B' hepatitis. At least two distinct viruses are involved. In industrialized countries approximately 90% of cases of post-transfusion hepatitis are caused by the hepatitis C virus (HCV), a small (30–60 nm), single-stranded RNA virus which may be related to the group B arboviruses (flaviviruses), which cause yellow fever, dengue and St. Louis encephalitis. The HCV genome has been cloned from the plasma of experimentally-infected chimpanzees and sequenced, but the agent has not yet been seen or cultured.

HCV infection is the most common cause of non-alcoholic liver disease in the USA; more than 150 000 cases of HCV infection occur every year. Approximately 75% of the cases are asymptomatic. Only 5–10% are associated with blood transfusions; about 40% are associated with intravenous drug use and 10% occur in homosexual men, heterosexual individuals with multiple sexual partners, or household or sexual contacts of patients with HCV infection. No source of infection can be identified in 40% of cases.

Anti-HCV antibody develops in only 60% of cases of acute HCV hepatitis, and appearance of antibody is often delayed for up to 6 months or a year after infection. Demonstration of anti-HCV is the only means presently available to confirm a diagnosis of HCV infection; whether or not clinically useful tests for detection of HCV antigen can be developed is not yet known.

Chronic liver disease develops in approximately 50% of individuals infected with the hepatitis C virus, and both cirrhosis and hepatocellular carcinoma are common sequelae. In recent studies approximately one-half of patients with chronic hepatitis C responded to administration of IFN_α, but relapse was frequent after discontinuation of therapy. Neither corticosteroids nor acyclovir are effective in treatment of chronic hepatitis C infection.

Epidemics of water-borne hepatitis in a number of countries, including India, Nepal, Myanmar, Pakistan, the USSR, Sudan, Somalia and Mexico, have been linked to an immunologically distinct virus, designated hepatitis E virus. This small (27–34 nm) single-stranded RNA virus is unrelated to HAV and the other picornaviruses, but may be related to the non-enveloped caliciviruses. It is present in the faeces of infected individuals, and has been demonstrated in hepatocytes of experimentally infected marmosets and *Cynomolgus* macaque monkeys. Hepatitis E virus appears to be one of the most common causes of acute hepatitis and jaundice in the Third World, but is rare in the USA and UK. Clinical hepatitis is observed more frequently in adults than in children.

The clinical illness produced by the hepatitis C and E viruses is usually mild, but there is a high case fatality rate in pregnant women who become infected with hepatitis E virus. Transient improvement followed by relapse is commonly seen in infection with hepatitis C virus. The incidence of fulminant hepatitis due to HCV appears to be low. The histopathological features are not always distinctive, but in some cases there is a disproportionate sinusoidal infiltrate and fat may be present (Fig. 5.12). Chronic hepatitis, which commonly

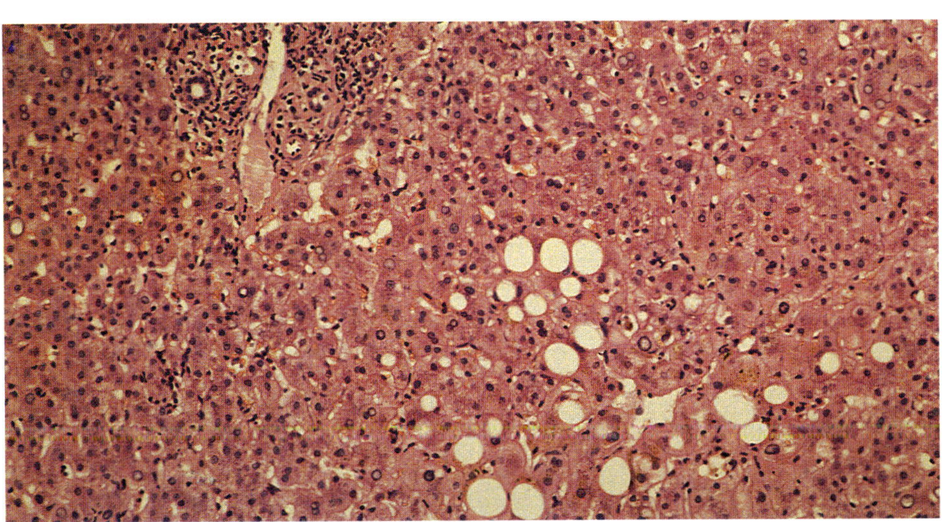

Fig. 5.12 Non-A, non-B hepatitis. Acute spotty hepatitis with macrovesicular fat in the centrilobular area, diffuse microvesicular fat and infiltration of inflammatory cells in the portal triad. By courtesy of Dr J. Newman.

follows infection with hepatitis C virus, is not seen in association with water-borne infections due to hepatitis E virus.

Hepatitis delta virus

The hepatitis delta virus (HDV) is a defective RNA virus which is capable of replication only during concomitant infection with HBV. Thus it occurs only in patients who have HB_sAg in the serum. It was discovered by immunofluorescent staining as a nuclear antigen distinct from the antigens of HBV, and is found in hepatocytes and serum of infected individuals. The hepatitis delta virus is a 35 nm particle which has an external coat of HB_sAg provided by the genome of HBV (the helper virus) and an internal delta antigen (HDV-Ag) provided by the genome of HDV. The genome of HDV is smaller than that of any animal virus, and resembles that of the viroids of plants.

The virus can cause either acute or chronic hepatitis. Acute delta hepatitis resembles other forms of acute hepatitis, but is more severe, with a case fatality rate of 2–20% (compared with less than 1% in acute hepatitis B). Chronic delta hepatitis is also more severe than other forms of chronic viral hepatitis; 70–80% of patients develop cirrhosis with portal hypertension. Acute delta hepatitis occurs as either coinfection or superinfection. Coinfection is the simultaneous occurrence of acute hepatitis B and acute delta infection. Superinfection is the occurrence of acute HDV infection in a chronic HBV carrier. Acute delta coinfection is usually mild and self limited, rarely leading to chronic hepatitis. In contrast, acute delta superinfection leads to chronic hepatitis in more than 80% of patients.

Diagnosis of delta hepatitis is made by detecting antibodies to HDV in the serum of a patient who has HB_sAg-positive hepatitis. Delta hepatitis should be suspected in any patient with acute or chronic hepatitis B infection, especially if the disease is severe or fulminant, or if the patient has a history of intravenous drug abuse or repeated exposure to blood or blood products. Clinical features suggesting delta infection are a biphasic illness in acute hepatitis or a history of jaundice or worsening of disease during the course of chronic hepatitis B infection.

Delta hepatitis occurs in three epidemiological settings. Endemic infection is especially common in the Mediterranean area and in the Middle East. The highest prevalence is reported from Kuwait and Saudi Arabia, where 20–40% of HB_sAg carriers have antibody to HDV. Delta hepatitis is rare in northern Europe, the USA and most of South America, and is also uncommon in southeast Asia and China, where the prevalence of chronic HBV infection is very high. The disease occurs in epidemic form in isolated populations in certain underdeveloped areas of the world, especially in northern South America and the Amazon Basin. In these outbreaks the disease is strikingly severe, with sudden onset of fulminant hepatitis and a rapidly fatal course. The epidemic form occurs most frequently in children. In northern Europe and the USA delta hepatitis occurs primarily in certain high risk groups, including intravenous drug addicts and patients who receive multiple blood transfusions or antihaemophilic globulin. Although sexual transmission of delta hepatitis can occur, it is rare in most but not all populations of male homosexuals.

Immunization against HBV infection also provides immunity against delta hepatitis. Unfortunately there is no way to prevent HDV superinfection in HB_sAg carriers, other than avoidance of contact. There is no established therapy for delta hepatitis. Corticosteroids are not effective in modifying the course or preventing progression of the disease. IFN_α inhibits replication of HDV and has produced clinical improvement in some patients, although discontinuation of therapy appears to be followed by relapse in nearly all cases. Results of liver transplantation in chronic delta hepatitis have been good, and some long-term survivors have remained both HB_sAg- and HDV-negative after transplantation.

Other Forms of Acute Hepatitis

Cytomegalovirus

Clinical hepatitis due to cytomegalovirus occurs mainly in immunocompromised patients, in whom the disease may be severe or even fatal. It is clinically indistinguishable from HBV hepatitis, but the histopathological picture is distinctive because of the intranuclear inclusions in giant cells produced by coalescence of proliferating bile duct epithelium, and infiltration of mononuclear cells (Fig. 5.13). Virus and antigens can be identified by culture or by immunofluorescent staining in blood and liver (Fig. 5.14), and in other body fluids and tissues.

Epstein–Barr virus

A mild, self-limited hepatitis, manifested by elevation of hepatocellular enzymes in the serum, occurs in 80–90% of patients with infectious mononucleosis due to the Epstein–Barr virus (Fig. 5.15). Occasionally severe hepatitis with jaundice is observed. Progression to chronic hepatitis or cirrhosis occurs rarely, if ever.

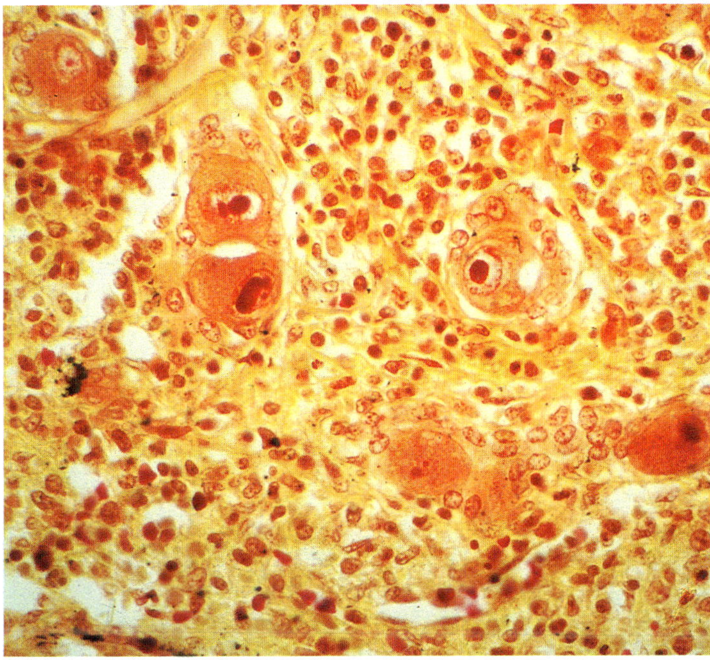

Fig. 5.13 Cytomegalovirus hepatitis. Histological section of liver, portal area, showing intranuclear inclusion bodies in giant cells formed from bile duct epithelial cells, with surrounding mononuclear cell infiltrate. Phloxine-tartrazine stain.

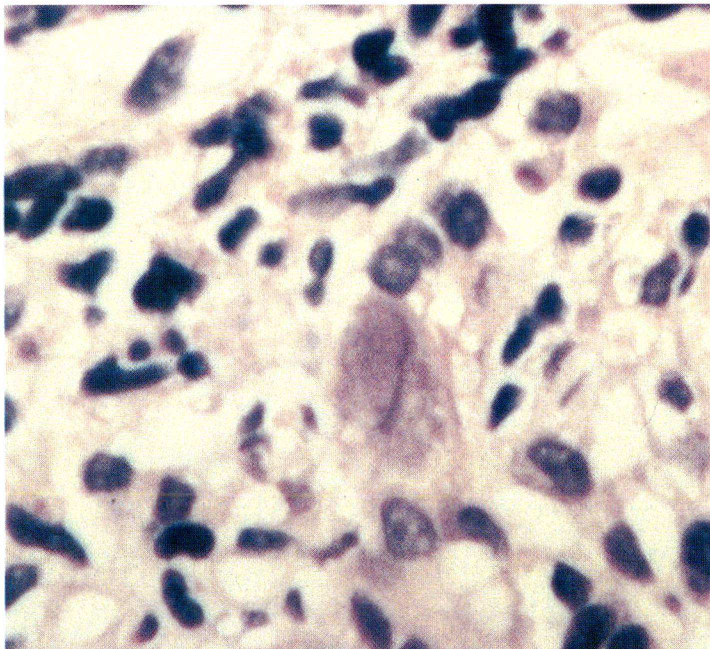

Fig. 5.14 Cytomegalovirus hepatitis: specific staining of CMV-infected giant cell using a DNA probe. By courtesy of Dr R. S. Markin.

Yellow Fever

Yellow fever is an acute viral illness caused by a group B arbovirus transmitted by the mosquito *Aedes aegypti*. The virus is viscerotropic and produces damage in the liver, kidney, heart and gastrointestinal tract. The name 'yellow fever' refers to the jaundice which is present in severe infections. After an incubation period of a few days the illness begins abruptly with fever and chills, headache, myalgias, nausea and vomiting and leucopenia. After a few days the patient appears to improve, but the illness returns with fever, jaundice, haemorrhages, albuminuria and renal failure. Death often occurs in 7–10 days, following a terminal stage characterized by agitation, delirium, shock and coma.

The hepatic lesion consists of acute coagulative necrosis of the midzonal portion of the lobule (Fig. 5.16). Intracellular hyaline deposits (Councilman bodies) and intranuclear eosinophilic inclusions (Torres bodies) may be seen. Even in severe cases there is a conspicuous absence of infiltration by inflammatory cells. Yellow fever formerly occurred throughout much of the world (except Asia), but is now found only in tropical America and Africa. Control of yellow fever has been achieved primarily by elimination of the insect vector from much of its former range, and the live attenuated 17D vaccine provides essentially life-long protection from infection.

Herpes simplex virus and varicella-zoster virus

In immunocompromised individuals with herpes simplex infection or varicella (chickenpox), the virus may disseminate to visceral organs, including the liver. The characteristic hepatic lesion is focal coagulative necrosis with little surrounding inflammation (Figs 5.17 & 5.18).

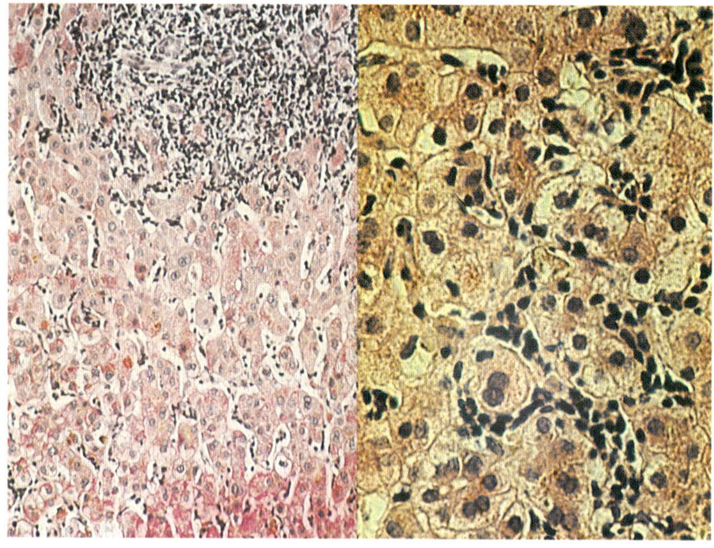

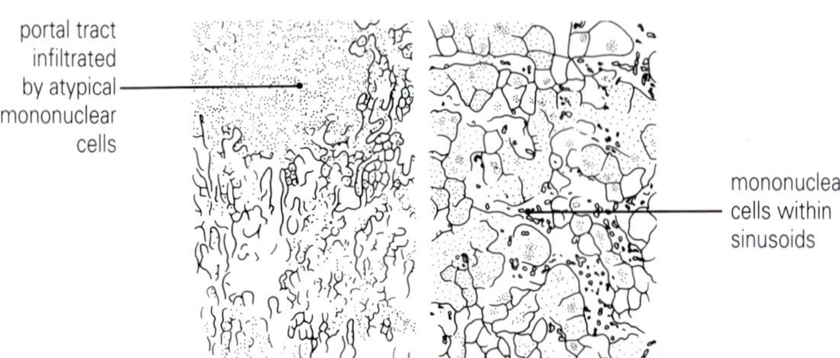

Fig. 5.15 Infectious mononucleosis. Histological sections of the liver. Left: A portal tract infiltrated by atypical mononuclear cells. By courtesy of Dr. I. Talbot. Right: Mononuclear cells extending into the sinusoids. H&E stain.

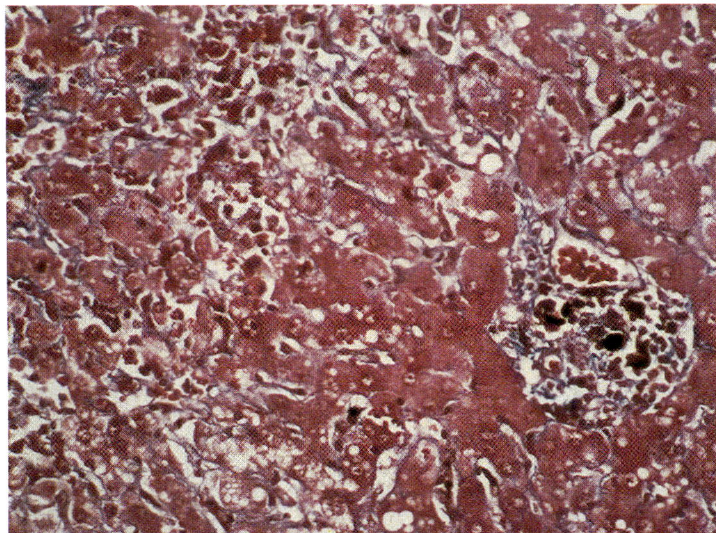

Fig. 5.16 Yellow fever. Histological section of liver showing the characteristic midzonal necrosis between central vein and portal tract. Masson trichrome stain.

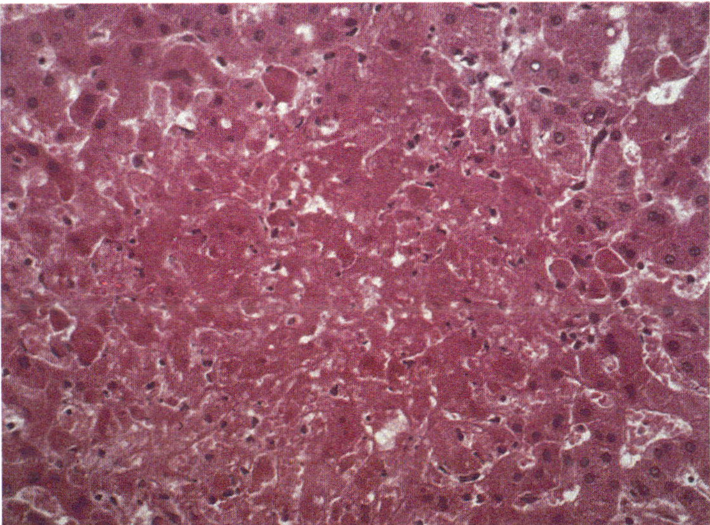

Fig. 5.17 Herpes simplex. Histological section of liver showing a necrotic focus with little surrounding inflammation. H&E stain.

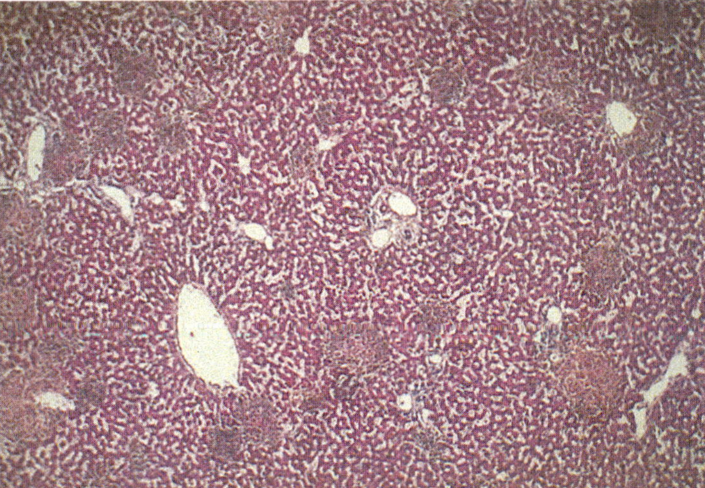

Fig. 5.18 Varicella. Histological section of liver showing necrotic foci. H&E stain. By courtesy of D. I. Talbot.

Q fever

In Q fever, a rickettsial disease, there may be hepatic necrosis and lipogranulomatous lesions with eosinophilic material surrounding the central vacuole (Fig. 5.19).

Syphilis

In congenital syphilis, there is a hepatitis characterized by fibrosis around individual hepatocytes (Fig. 5.20), and there are abundant spirochaetes in the liver. In tertiary syphilis the typical lesion is the

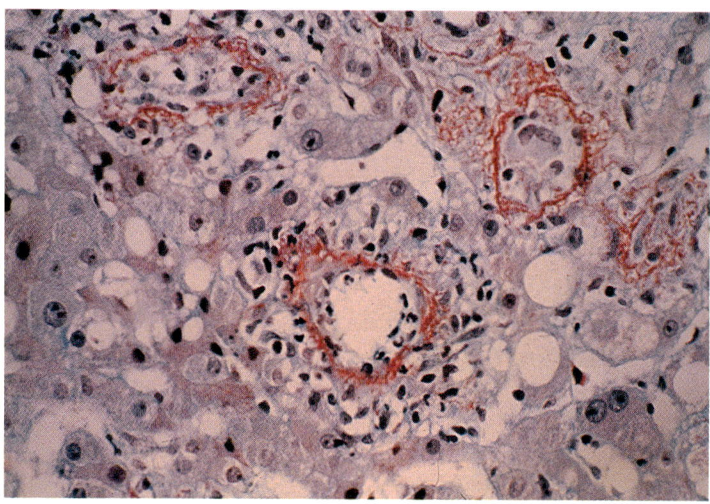

Fig. 5.19 Q fever. Histological section of liver showing the characteristic lipogranulomatous-like lesion – a granuloma with a central vacuole and a red 'fibrinoid' rim. Martius scarlet blue stain.

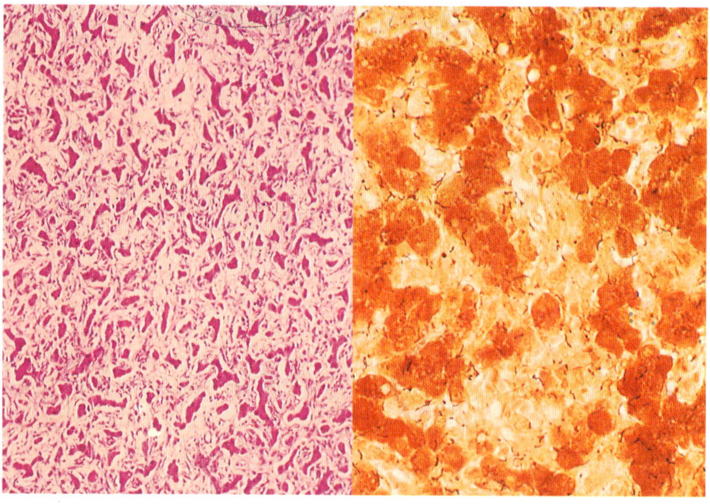

Fig. 5.20 Congenital syphilis. Histological sections of liver showing diffuse pericellular fibrosis (left, H&E stain) and spirochaetes (right, Levaditi stain). By courtesy of Dr I. Talbot.

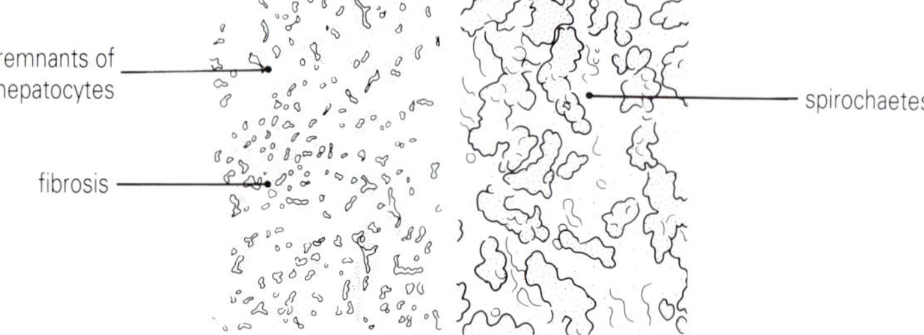

gumma, a necrotic nodule surrounded by granulation tissue (Fig. 5.21), which produces deep scars (hepar lobatum) as it heals by fibrosis.

Leptospirosis

Most infections with *Leptospira* species are either asymptomatic or result in mild anicteric infections without evidence of significant hepatic involvement. In severe cases of leptospirosis (Weil's disease), jaundice and impaired liver function are characteristically present. The jaundice is usually not associated with hepatocellular necrosis and leptospires are rarely seen in the liver (Fig. 5.22). After recovery, hepatic function returns to normal.

Severe bacterial infection

Jaundice is a well-recognized complication of severe bacterial infection in newborns, but this syndrome occurs rarely in adults. Occasionally in severe bacteraemic infections, especially those due to *Escherichia coli* and related members of the family Enterobacteriaceae, cholestatic jaundice is observed. Serum bilirubin and alkaline phosphatase levels are elevated, but transaminases are usually normal or elevated only slightly. Histopathological examination reveals intrahepatic cholestasis with little or no hepatocellular necrosis.

Reye's syndrome

Reye's syndrome is a syndrome of unknown aetiology seen primarily in children following influenza B (less commonly influenza A), varicella and a number of other viral infections. The incidence appears to be increased in children who have received aspirin. Involvement of the central nervous system is the most serious aspect of Reye's syndrome, and most deaths are due to cerebral oedema. In the liver the predominant findings are fatty infiltration of hepatocytes, with multiple small

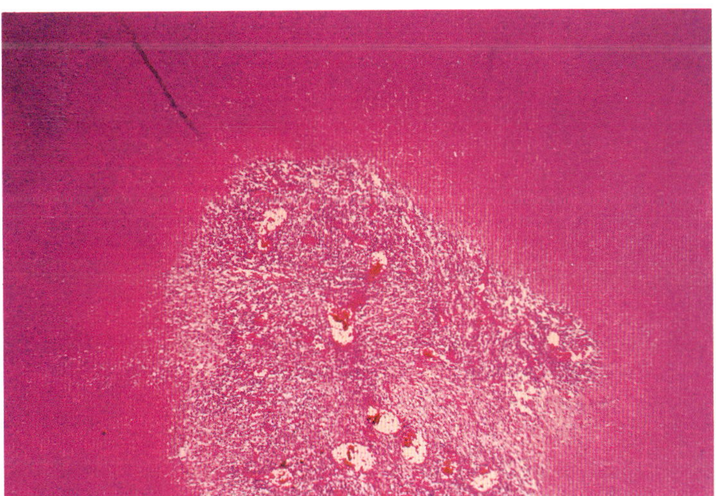

Fig. 5.21 Tertiary syphilis. Histological section of liver showing a gumma. H&E stain. By courtesy of Dr I. Talbot.

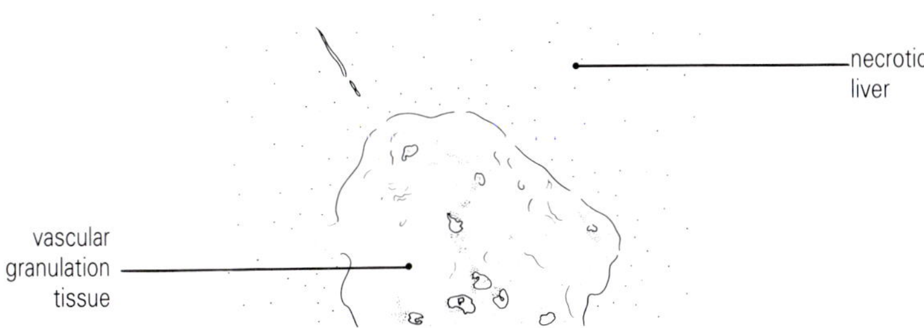

droplets of lipids uniformly distributed throughout the cells (Figs 5.23 and 5.24). Swelling and pleomorphism of hepatic mitochondria are seen using electron microscopy. Inflammatory changes are absent, and there is little or no hepatocellular necrosis.

GRANULOMATOUS HEPATITIS

Formation of granulomas in the liver is observed in a wide variety of diseases, both infectious and non-infectious. The essential event in granuloma

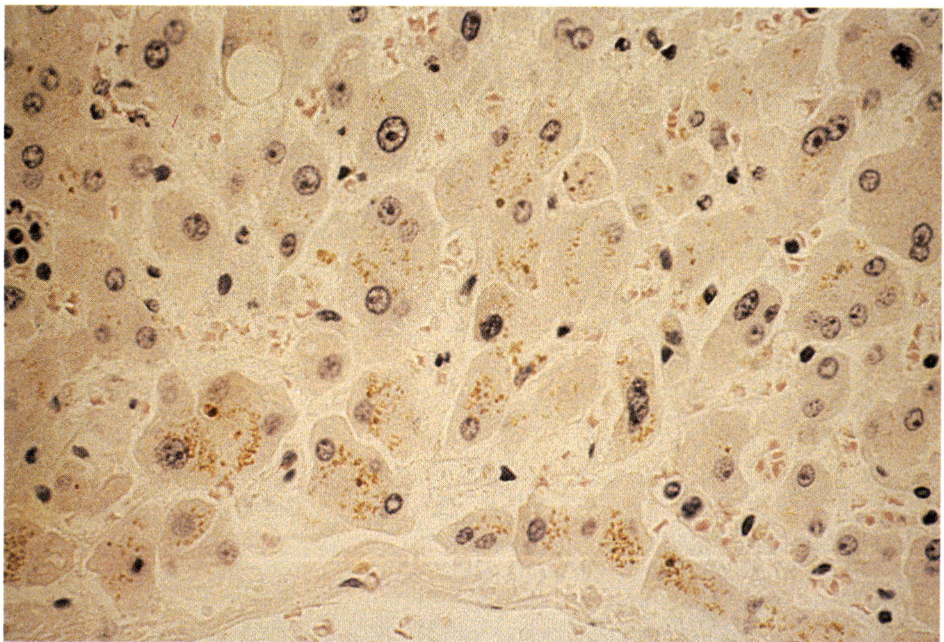

Fig. 5.22 Leptospirosis: Hepatocytes contain large amounts of bilirubin. There are scattered lymphocytes and numerous irregularly-shaped nuclear fragments. By courtesy of Dr J. Newman.

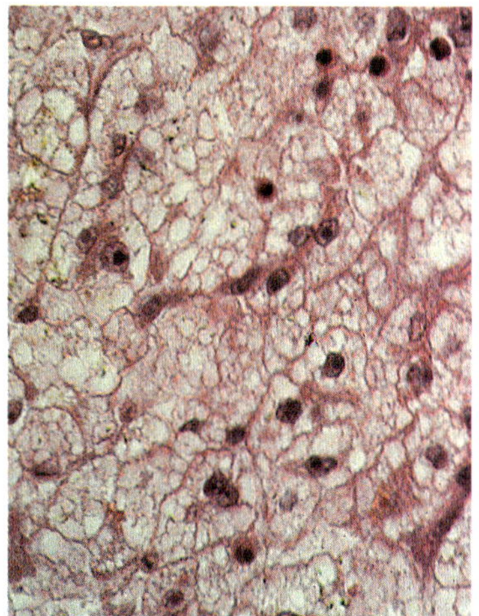

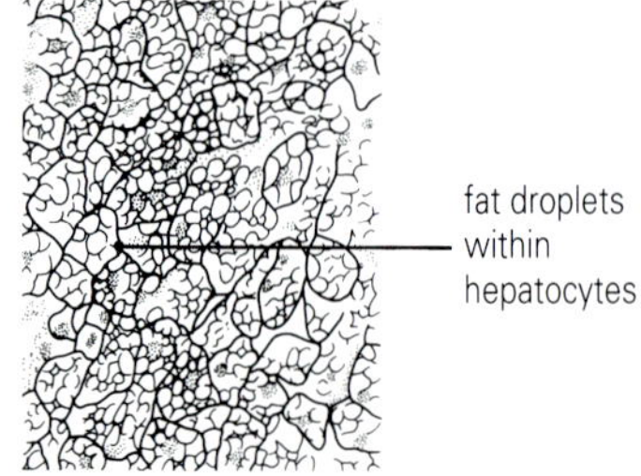

Fig. 5.23 Reye's syndrome: Histological section of liver showing fat within cytoplasmic microvesicles. H&E stain. Courtesy of Dr I. Talbot.

formation is the transformation of the monocyte/macrophage into an epithelioid cell. This event is stimulated by the presence of antigen, either soluble or particulate (e.g. microorganisms and/or their products) in a sensitized cell.

Tuberculosis

The most common infectious disease associated with granuloma formation in the liver is tuberculosis.

Outside the liver, tuberculous granulomas usually exhibit caseation necrosis, but hepatic granulomas due to tuberculosis are characteristically noncaseating (Fig. 5.25). Hepatic granulomas are present in more than 90% of patients with miliary tuberculosis, but are also extremely prevalent in pulmonary and in other extrapulmonary forms of the disease (70–80%). Tubercle bacilli can be demonstrated either by staining techniques or culture in approximately half of patients with miliary

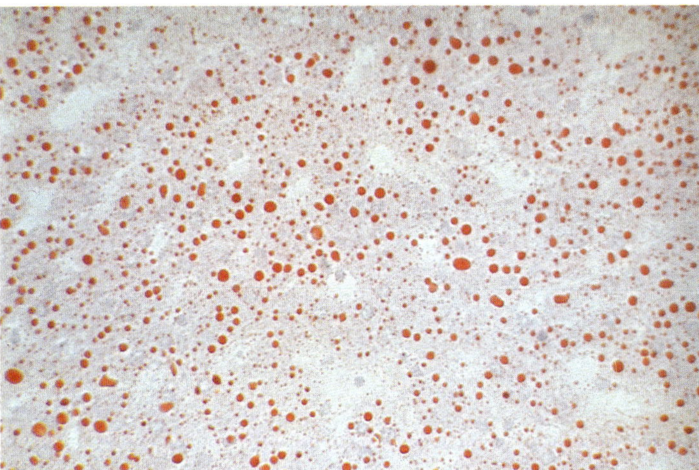

Fig. 5.24 Reye's syndrome. Liver section with fat globules stained by oil red O. By courtesy of Dr I. Talbot.

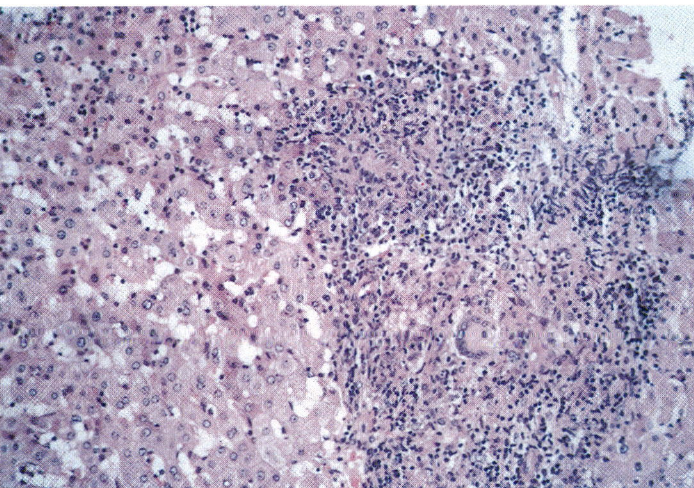

Fig. 5.25 Miliary tuberculosis. Liver biopsy showing two contiguous tubercles and epithelioid cells, a few Langhans-type giant cells and lymphocytes. There is no caseation. H&E stain.

tuberculosis (Fig. 5.26), but are detected much less frequently in the granulomas associated with other forms of tuberculosis.

Mycobacterial infections in AIDS

Infections due to *Mycobacterium tuberculosis* and *M. avium–intracellulare* are very common in patients with AIDS. Most AIDS patients with tuberculosis have disseminated or other extrapulmonary forms of the disease, and lesions are commonly found in the liver. Sometimes typical granulomas are found, but often the granulomas are poorly formed or the lesions are abscesses rather than granulomas. Infection with *M. avium–intracellulare* usually occurs late in the course of AIDS, in patients who

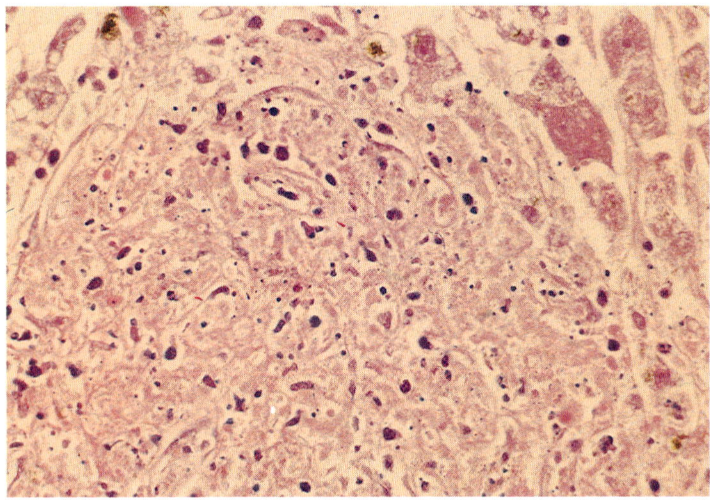

Fig. 5.26 Miliary tuberculosis. Acid-fast stain of hepatic granuloma showing a few red-staining tubercle bacilli. By courtesy of Dr T. Gramlich.

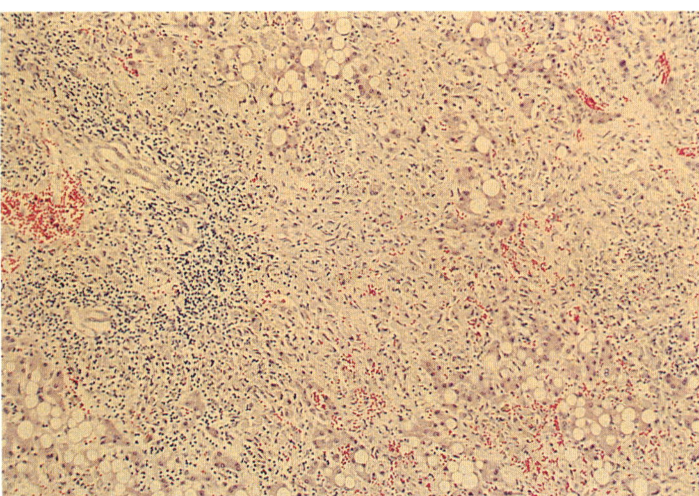

Fig. 5.27 Disseminated infection due to *M. avium–intracellulare*: Poorly formed granuloma in the liver of a patient with AIDS. By courtesy of Dr T. Gramlich.

are profoundly immunocompromised. In such patients granulomas are poorly formed or absent (Fig. 5.27).

Disseminated fungal infection

Disseminated fungal infections are also commonly associated with granulomas in the liver. In the USA, disseminated histoplasmosis is the most common fungal infection associated with hepatic granulomas (Fig. 5.28), and liver biopsy is a valuable technique in the diagnosis of this infection (Fig. 5.29) and in the diagnosis of disseminated African histoplasmosis (Fig. 5.30). Hepatic candidiasis appears to be increasing in frequency among patients with cancer (Fig. 5.31); in these patients the lesions

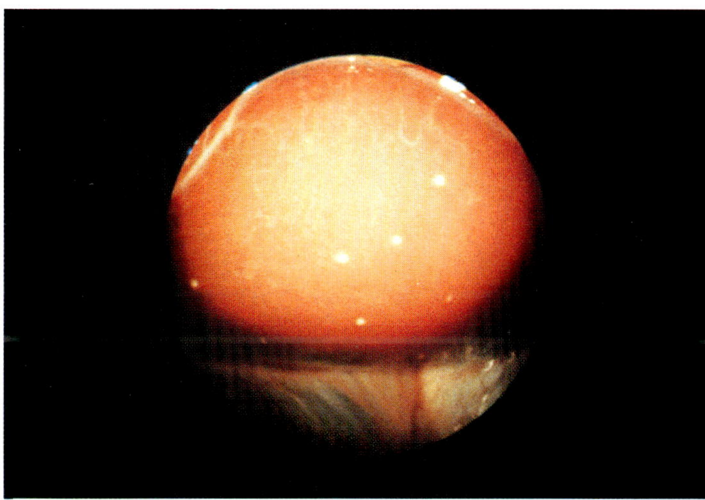

Fig. 5.28 Histoplasmosis. Laparoscopic view of the surface of the liver showing healed granulomatous lesions in a patient with old, healed histoplasmosis. Biopsy of the lesions revealed calcification. By courtesy of Dr J. T. Cunningham.

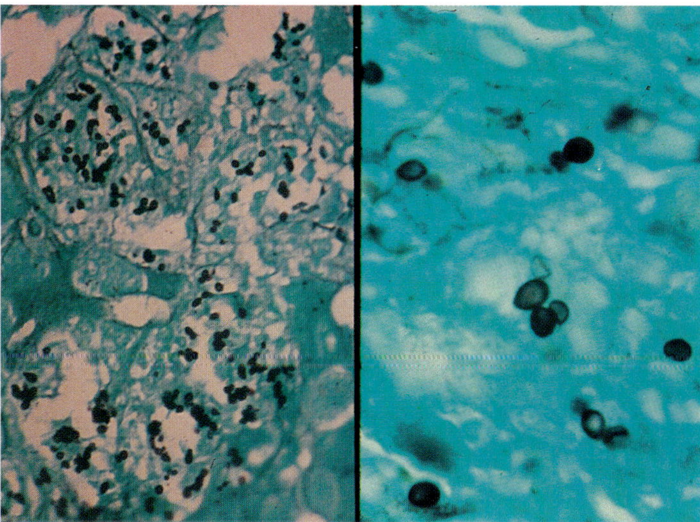

Fig. 5.29 Disseminated histoplasmosis. Left: Upper section of liver showing yeast forms of *Histoplasma capsulatum* in hepatic sinusoids. Right: Yeast forms of *H. capsulatum* from a lesion of the vocal cord. Gomori-methenamine silver stains. By courtesy of Dr H. P. Holley, Jr.

often resemble abscesses rather than granulomas. Hepatic involvement is occasionally seen during systemic infection with a wide variety of other fungal organisms including *Cryptococcus neoformans* (Fig. 5.32).

Schistosomiasis

The adult trematode worms *Schistosoma mansoni* and *S. japonicum* (see also Chapter 3) reside in the portal and mesenteric veins, and granulomas surrounding the eggs of these organisms may occur in the liver (Fig. 5.33). If infection is extensive, portal hypertension, hepatosplenomegaly and oesophageal varices may result.

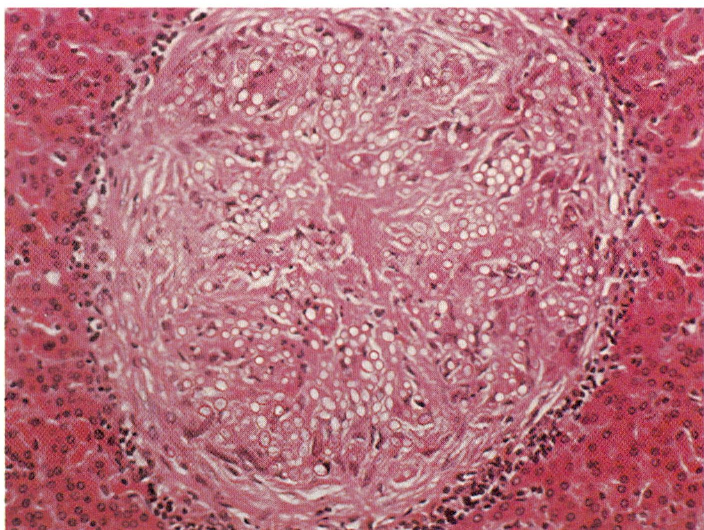

Fig. 5.30 Histoplasmosis. Hepatic granuloma in African histoplasmosis, showing round vacuolated *H. duboisii* organisms. H&E stain.

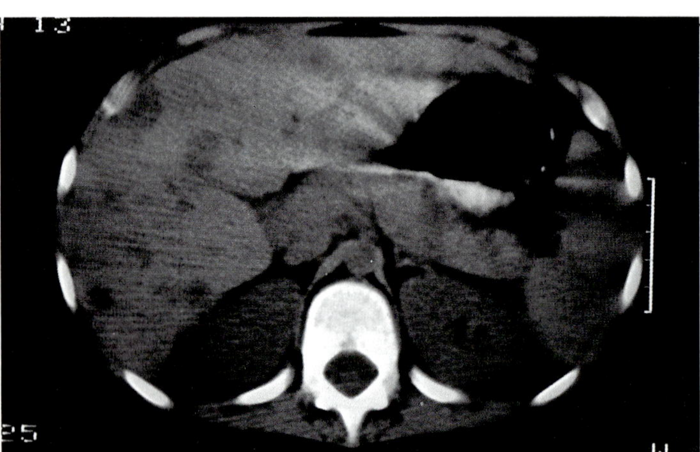

Fig. 5.31 Disseminated candidiasis. CT scan showing multiple hepatosplenic abscesses in a patient with leukaemia. By courtesy of Dr C. Kibbler.

Leishmaniasis

Extensive liver involvement may also occur in visceral leishmaniasis (kala-azar). In this disease there is marked proliferation of Kupffer cells, many of which are filled with the amastigote forms of *Leishmania donovani* (Fig. 5.34).

Other causes

Other infectious diseases in which liver granulomas are sometimes observed include toxoplasmosis, visceral larva migrans, Q fever (see Fig. 5.19), cat scratch disease, CMV infection, hepatitis B, and infectious mononucleosis.

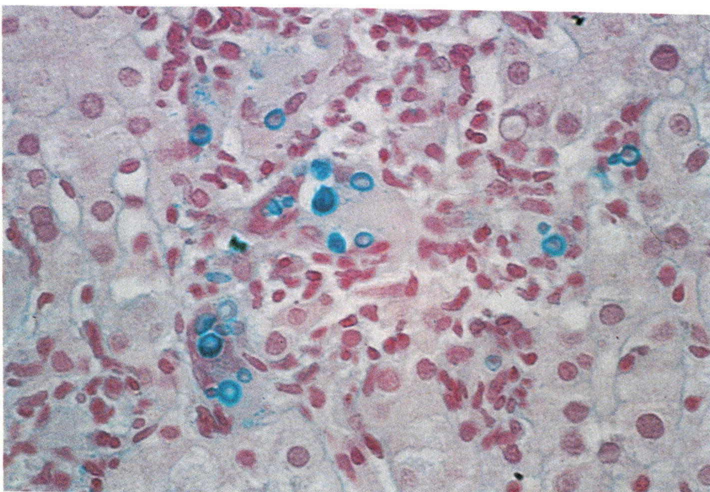

Fig. 5.32 Cryptococcosis. Histological section of liver showing cryptococci staining blue with alcian blue stain.

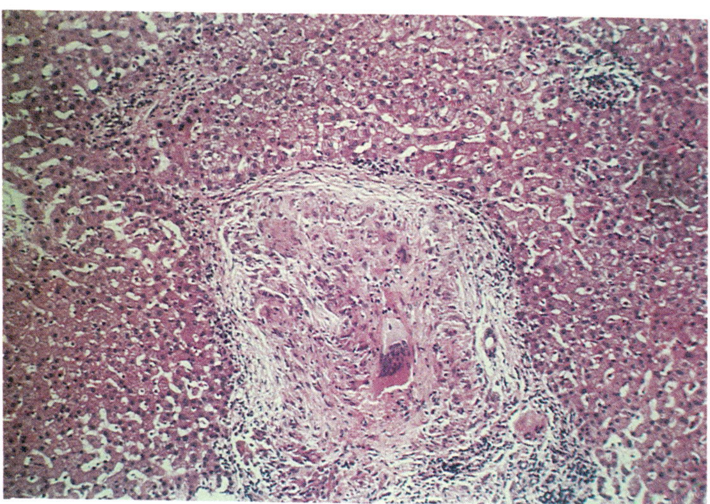

Fig. 5.33 Schistosomiasis. Eggs of *S. mansoni* in liver with surrounding granulomatous reaction. H&E stain.

Non-infectious granulomatous diseases

Sarcoidosis is the non-infectious disease most commonly associated with hepatic granulomas. In sarcoidosis and in other non-infectious causes of hepatic granuloma formation, the granulomas are non-caseating (Fig. 5.35). Hepatic granulomas are also seen in Hodgkin's disease and in various hypersensitivity states such as erythema nodosum. In approximately 50% of patients with granulomas in the liver, the lesions appear to be limited to the liver and no cause can be found. Presence of extensive granuloma formation in the liver is often associated with fever, and this condition is a common cause of 'fever of undetermined origin'.

HEPATIC ABSCESS

Abscesses in the liver may be due to *Entamoeba histolytica* or to various bacterial organisms. Clinical

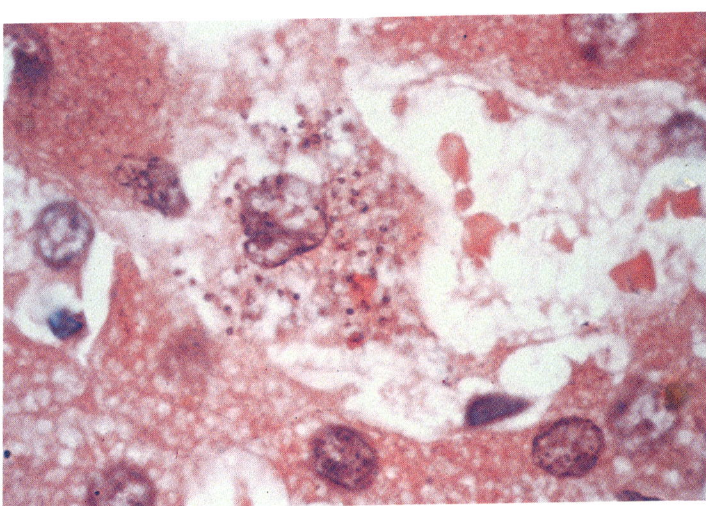

Fig. 5.34 Visceral leishmaniasis (kala-azar). Section of liver showing a mononuclear phagocytic cell in a sinusoid containing many amastigote forms of *L. donovani*. H&E stain.

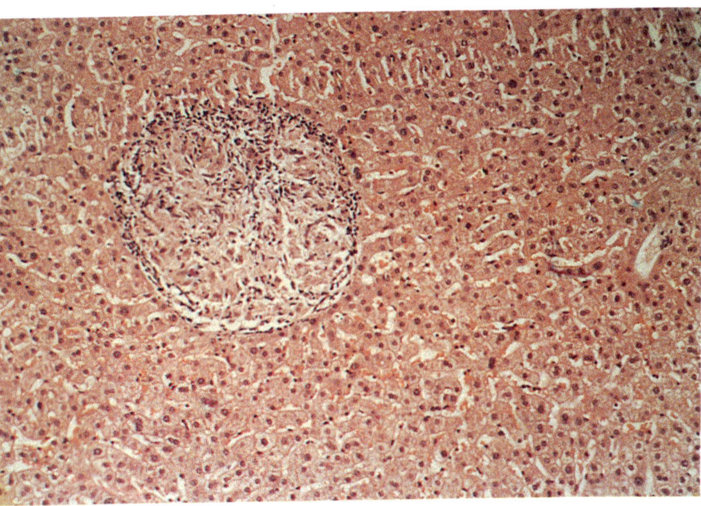

Fig. 5.35 Sarcoidosis. Histological section showing a discrete non-caseating granuloma in the liver, composed primarily of epithelioid cells, surrounded by a thin rim of lymphocytes. H&E stain.

differentiation between the two types on the basis of such features as body temperature, leucocytosis or local pain and tenderness is notoriously unreliable.

Amoebic abscesses

Amoebic liver abscesses are characteristically single and located in the right lobe and may be extremely large (Figs 5.36 & 5.37). Most patients do not give a history consistent with preceding or current amoebic dysentery. An enlarged, tender liver, elevated diaphragm on chest x-ray, leucocytosis and elevated serum alkaline phosphatase levels are usually observed. Radioisotope scanning, computed tomography and ultrasonography are valuable for demonstrating the abscess. A serological test for amoebiasis is almost always positive in amoebic liver abscess. Occasionally, multiple amoebic abscesses are present (Fig. 5.38). The abscess cavities contain

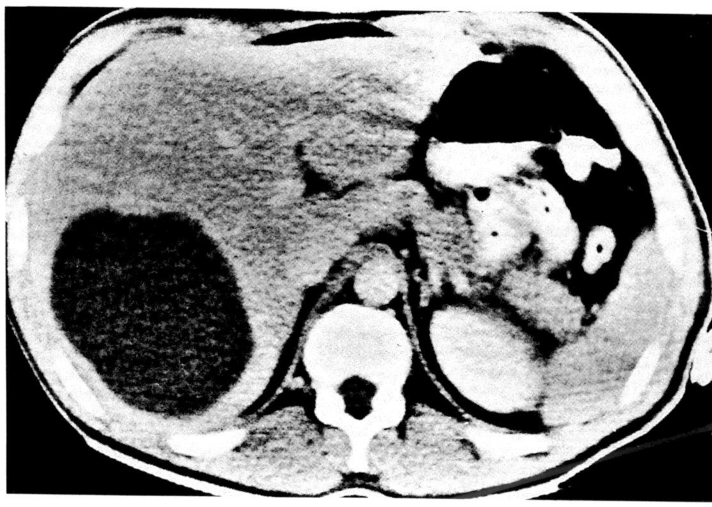

Fig. 5.36 Amoebic liver abscess. CT scan showing large single amoebic abscess in the right lobe of the liver. Courtesy of Dr F. Pittman.

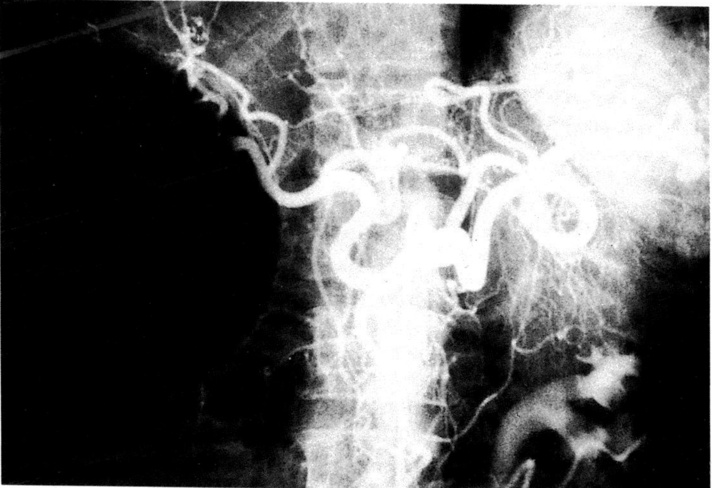

Fig. 5.37 Amoebic liver abscess. Coeliac angiogram showing absence of vascular structures in a large amoebic liver abscess. The liquified necrotic material has been aspirated from the abscess and replaced by air. Courtesy of Dr J. Cunningham.

whitish, incompletely liquified, necrotic material which is sharply distinct from the normal liver tissue, and thick, brownish, odourless, liquified material consisting of necrotic liver tissue, inflammatory cells, and small or large numbers of amoebae (Figs 5.39 & 5.40). This material is regarded by some as resembling anchovy paste. Medical therapy with metronidazole or other drugs is usually effective and surgical drainage is rarely required.

Bacterial abscesses

Bacterial liver abscesses may occur secondary to nearby infection in the biliary tract, or the organisms may reach the liver via the portal vein (from intra-abdominal infections such as appendiceal abscess) or the systemic circulation. They are more likely than amoebic abscesses to be multiple. If the source of the abscess is infection in the biliary tract,

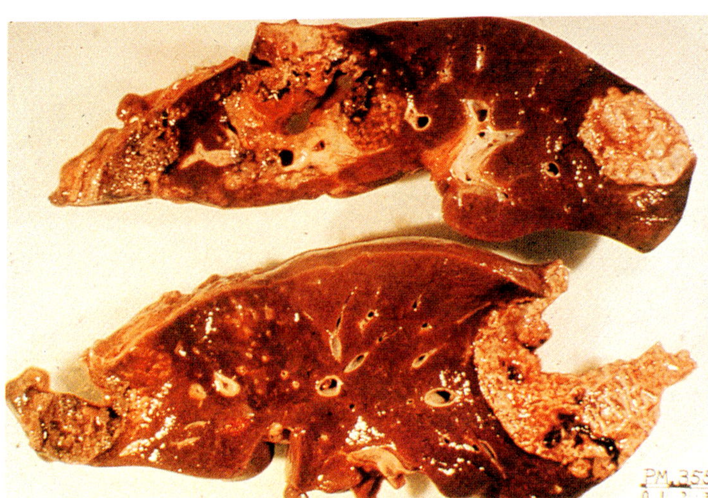

Fig. 5.38 Amoebic liver abscess. Cut surface of liver showing multiple amoebic abscesses. Note the large central abscess containing 'anchovy paste' material and thick irregular lining of abscess cavities, composed of necrotic liver which has not yet liquified. Courtesy of Dr J. T. Galambos.

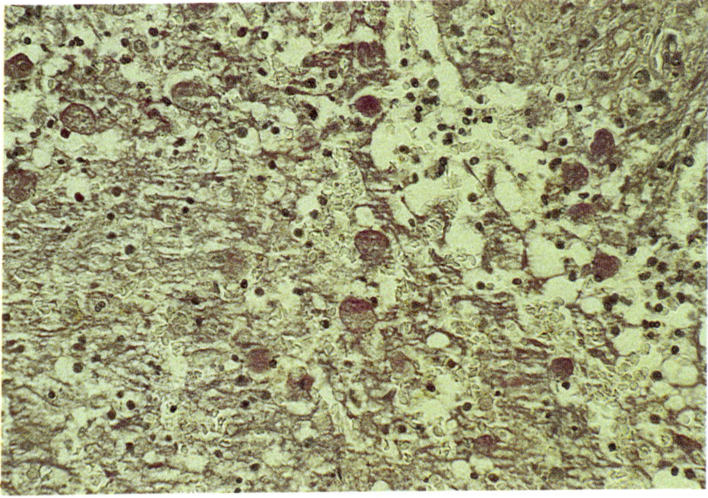

Fig. 5.39 Amoebic liver abscess. Trophozoites of *Entamoeba histolytica* in necrotic liver tissue. By courtesy of Dr C. Edwards.

the most common aetiological agents are *E. coli* and other members of the Enterobacteriaceae, including salmonella. If the infection has reached the liver via the portal vein, anaerobic bacteria, with or without aerobic species, are usually found. Streptococci of the *S. intermedius* (*S. milleri*) group are found in up to 80% of the lesions. Radionuclide scanning (Fig. 5.41), computed

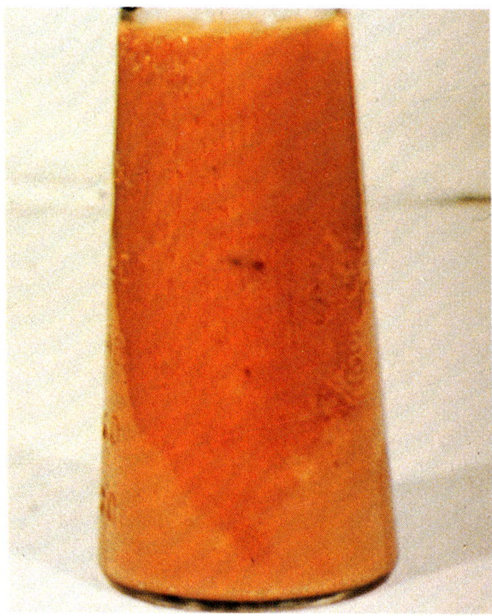

Fig. 5.40 Amoebic liver abscess. 'Anchovy paste' material aspirated from an amoebic abscess of the liver. This fluid, unlike that found in pyogenic liver abscess, is odourless. Amoebae may or may not be readily found upon microscopic examination. By courtesy of Dr K. Juniper.

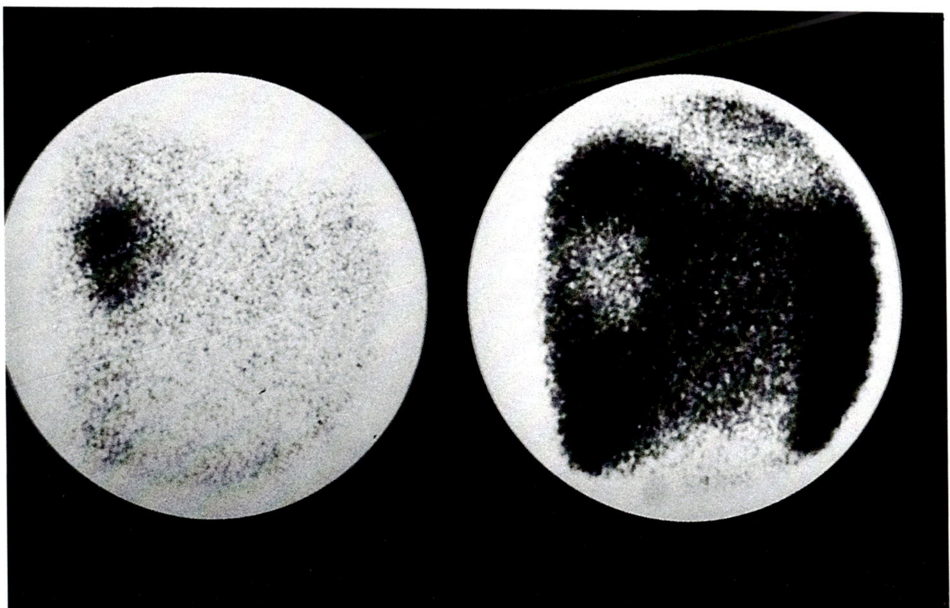

Fig. 5.41 Pyogenic liver abscess. Gallium (left) and technetium (right) radionuclide scans of the liver. Gallium is picked up by inflammatory cells in the wall and cavity of the abscess, and thus outlines the abscess itself. Technetium is deposited in the Kuppfer cells of normally functioning liver, so activity is absent from the area involved by abscess. By courtesy of Dr. H. P. Holley, Jr.

tomographic scanning (Figs 5.42 & 5.43) and ultrasonography (Fig. 5.44) are valuable for confirming the presence of suspected liver abscesses. Percutaneous catheter drainage, using computed tomography to achieve precise placement of the catheter (Fig. 5.45), has obviated the need for surgical drainage in most cases of bacterial liver abscess. When multiple abscesses are present it may be necessary to drain several of the largest cavities. Treatment with an antibiotic effective against the infecting organisms should be administered for from one to several months. Amoebic liver abscesses are sometimes secondarily infected with bacteria; this type of combined infection may be very difficult to diagnose.

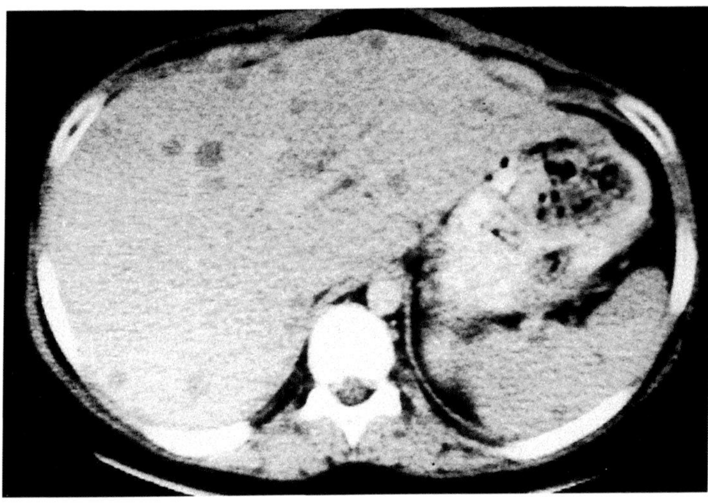

Fig. 5.42 Pyogenic liver abscess. CT scan showing multiple liver abscesses due to *Pseudomonas aeruginosa* in a severely neutropenic patient with chronic aplastic anaemia. By courtesy of D. N. Holland.

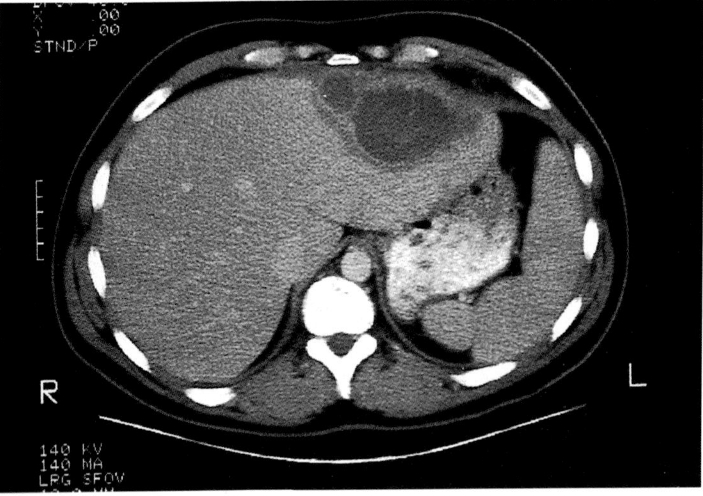

Fig. 5.43 Pyogenic liver abscess. CT scan showing a large abscess in the left lobe of the liver, with septum formation between compartments of the abscess. By courtesy of Dr R. Noble.

ECHINOCOCCOSIS (HYDATID DISEASE)

Adults of the dog tapeworm, *Echinococcus granulosus*, inhabit the intestinal tract of dogs.

Sheep and cattle ingest the cysts in food contaminated by canine faeces. The cysts dissolve in the stomach and the liberated ova penetrate the intestinal wall. Dogs become infected by eating the vis-

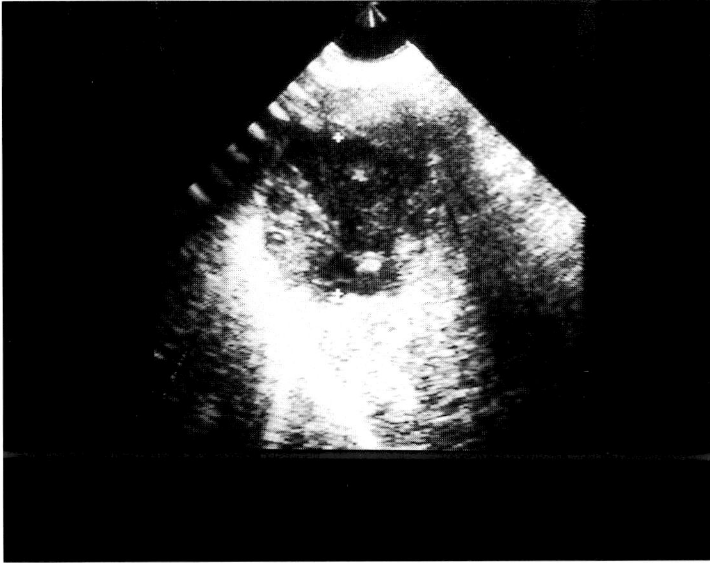

Fig. 5.44 Pyogenic liver abscess. Ultrasound scan showing large intrahepatic abscess, with incomplete septum formation within the abscess cavity. By courtesy of Dr R. Noble.

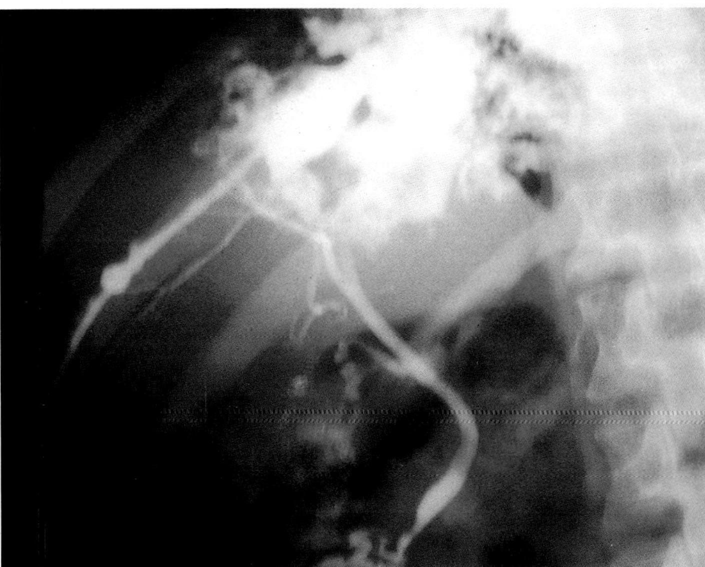

Fig. 5.45 Pyogenic liver abscess. Percutaneous drainage of liver abscess. Injection of contrast material to delineate extent of abscess formation.

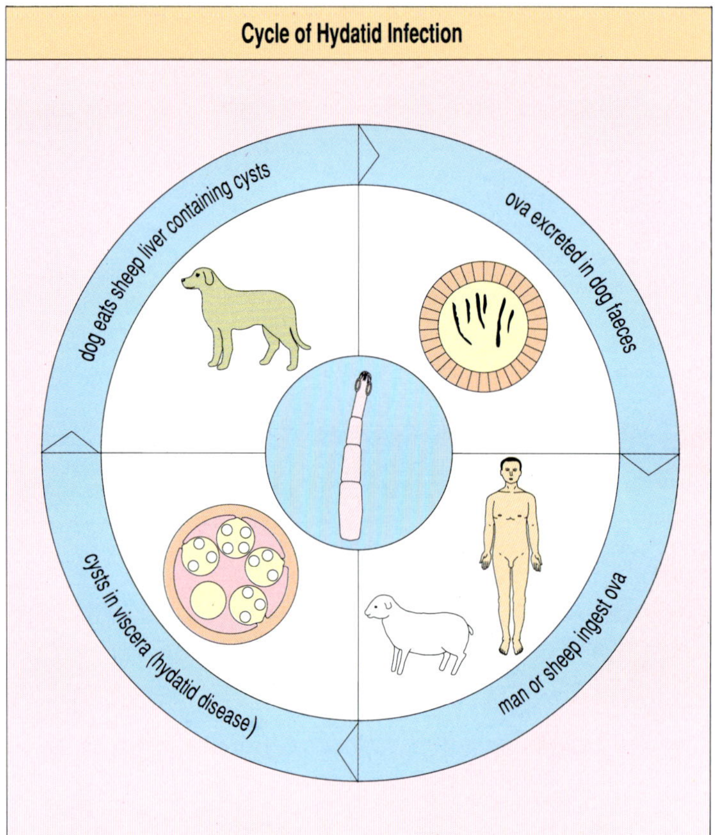

Fig. 5.46 The cycle of *Echinococcus* (hydatid infection).

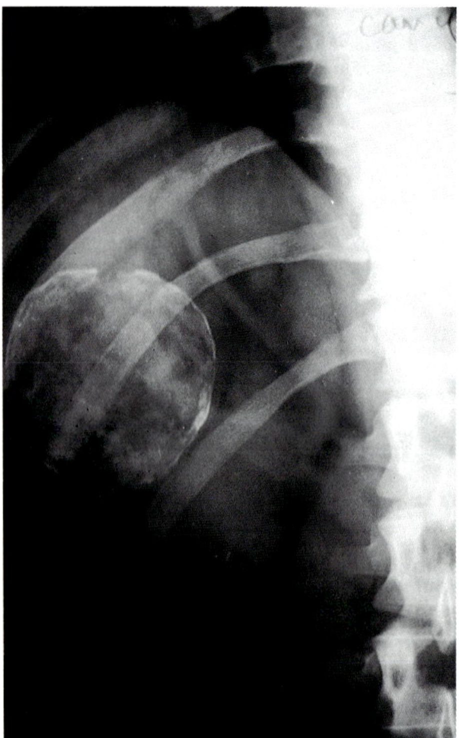

Fig. 5.47 Echinococcosis. Abdominal radiograph showing a calcified hydatid cyst in the liver.

cera of dead, infected sheep and cattle, and the cycle is maintained (Fig. 5.46). Man is an accidental dead-end host, infected by contact with contaminated dog faeces, and plays no role in the cycle of infection. After penetrating the bowel wall the embryos travel via the portal blood to the liver and other organs. They may die and calcify (Fig. 5.47) or they may slowly enlarge over many years, producing disease by pressure effects or rupturing into the peritoneal cavity or pleural space with dissemination of the larvae (scolices) and production of multiple new lesions (Figs 5.48, 5.49 & 5.50).

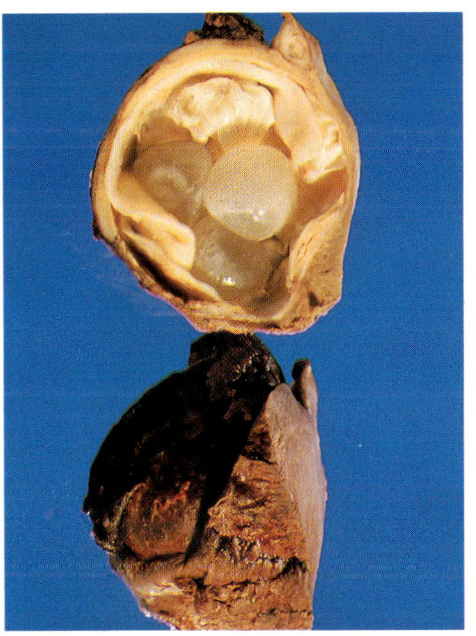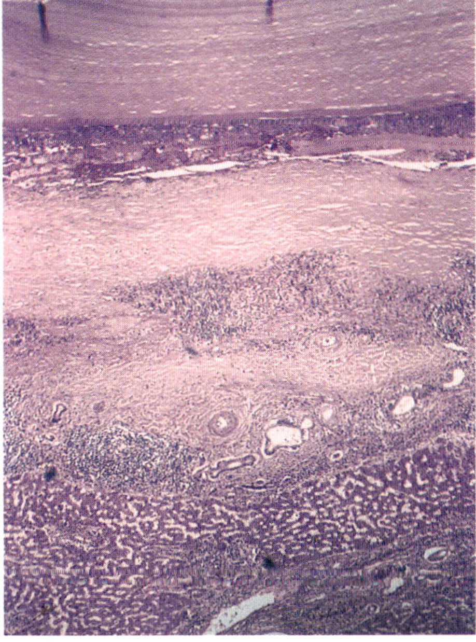

Fig. 5.48 Echinococcosis. Left: An echinococcal cyst showing daughter cysts, resected from the liver. Right: Histological section showing the layers of an hydatid cyst. H&E stain.

The cysts can be visualized by ultrasonography (Fig. 5.51), CT scanning (Fig. 5.52) or other imaging techniques (Fig. 5.53), and serological tests may provide a specific aetiological diagnosis. In cases where treatment is required, surgical removal, marsupialization and sterilization of cyst contents with formalin, hypertonic sodium chloride or iodine solution, or therapy with antihelminthic agents such as mebendazole, albendazole or praziquantel, may be effective. Infection in dogs can be prevented by proper disposal of sheep and cattle carcasses.

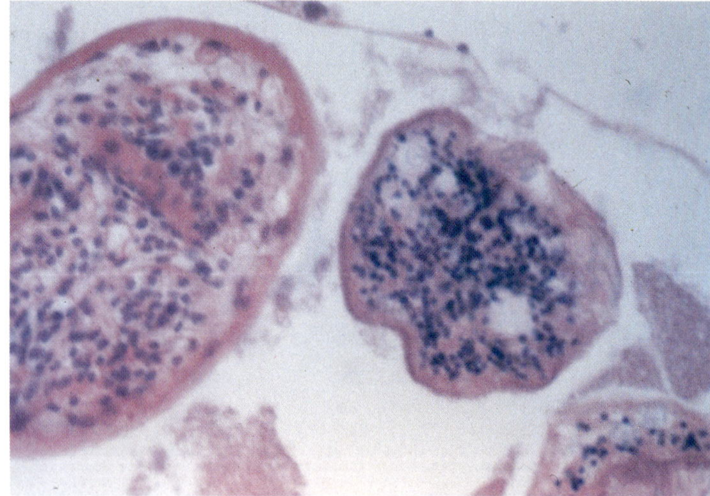

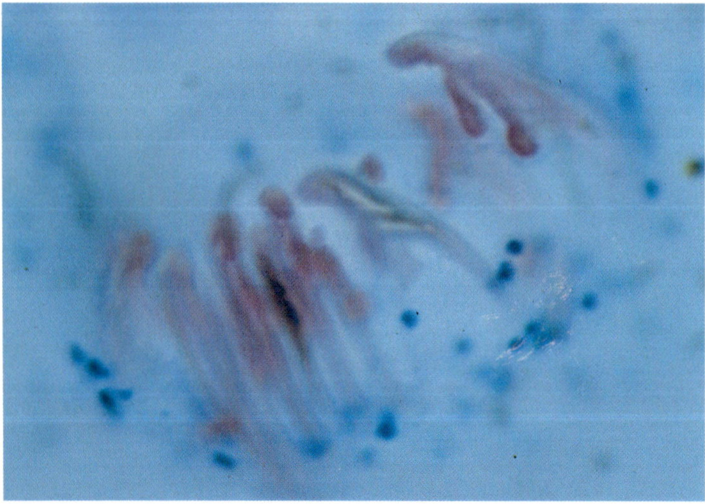

Fig. 5.49 Echinococcosis. Top: Scolices of *E. granulosus*. H&E stain. Bottom: Hooklet at a higher magnification. Ziehl-Neelsen stain.

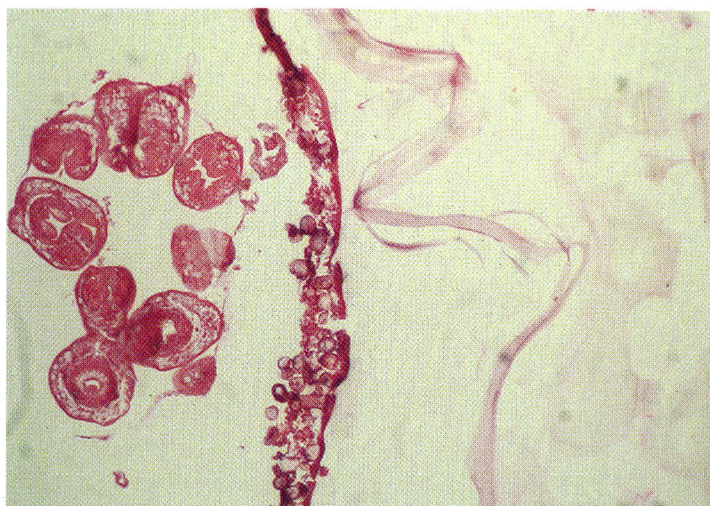

Fig. 5.50 Echinococcosis. Cyst in liver showing (from right) laminated, non-nuclear layer, nucleated germinal layer with many brood capsules attached, and multiple scolices within the cyst cavity. By courtesy of Dr C. Edwards.

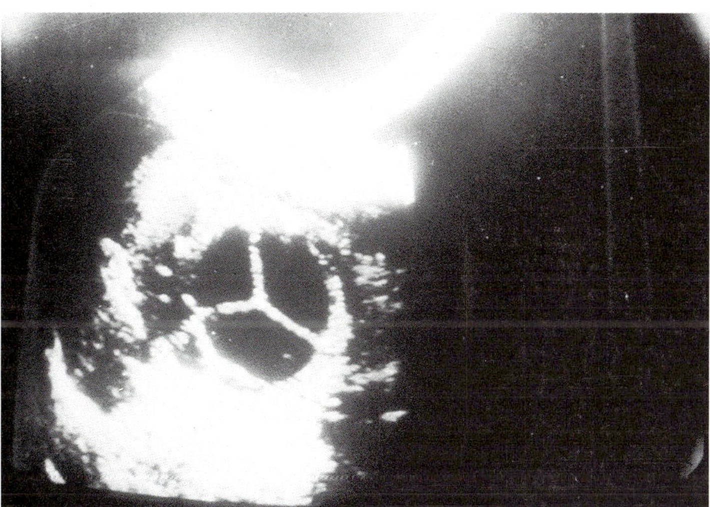

Fig. 5.51 Echinococcosis. Ultrasound scan showing multiloculated cyst in liver.

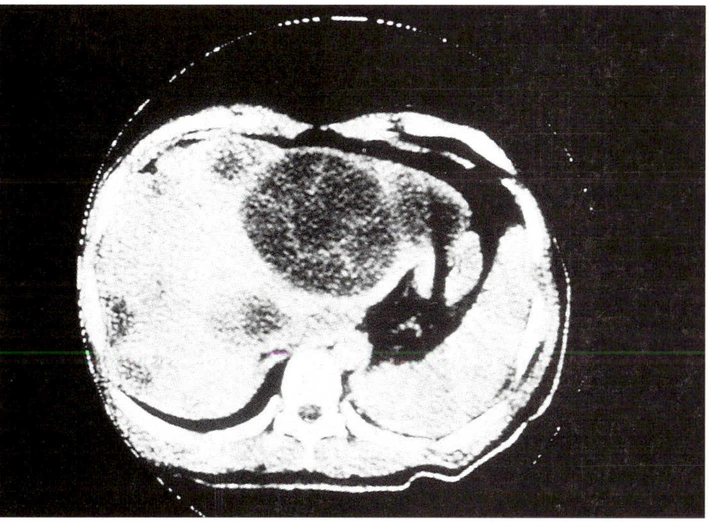

Fig. 5.52 Echinococcosis. CT scan showing large multiloculated cyst in left lobe of liver.

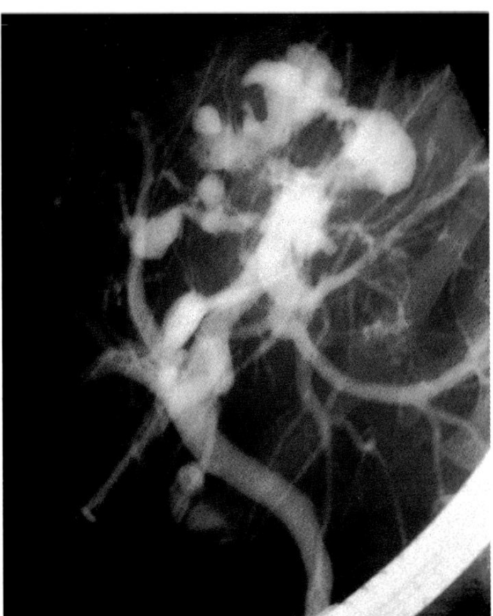

Fig. 5.53 Echinococcosis. Endoscopic retrograde cholangio-pancreatography (ERCP) showing intrahepatic hydatid cystic spaces draining into the biliary tree.

Chapter 6

Infections of the Biliary Tract

CHOLECYSTITIS

Infection of the gallbladder (cholecystitis) may be acute or chronic, or the two types may coexist. In more than 90% of cases, stones are present in the cystic duct. Common clinical findings include pain in the right upper quadrant of the abdomen, fever, jaundice and a palpable gallbladder. Ultrasonography (Fig. 6.1) and hepatobiliary radionuclide scanning with an acetanilide iminodiacetic acid (IDA) derivative are both rapid and sensitive techniques for diagnosing this disease. The causative bacteria are most commonly *E. coli* and other organisms of the family Enterobacteriaceae, and streptococci. Anaerobic bacteria are found occasionally, but seem to be involved less frequently than in most other types of intra-abdominal infection.

In acute cholecystitis (Figs 6.2 & 6.3) there is an intense acute inflammatory reaction which may involve the full thickness of the gallbladder wall and may progress to transmural necrosis and perforation. In emphysematous cholecystitis, a severe form occurring primarily in diabetics, gas may be seen within the lumen and wall of the gallbladder (Fig. 6.4). In chronic cholecystitis, the wall of the gallbladder may be markedly thickened; multiple

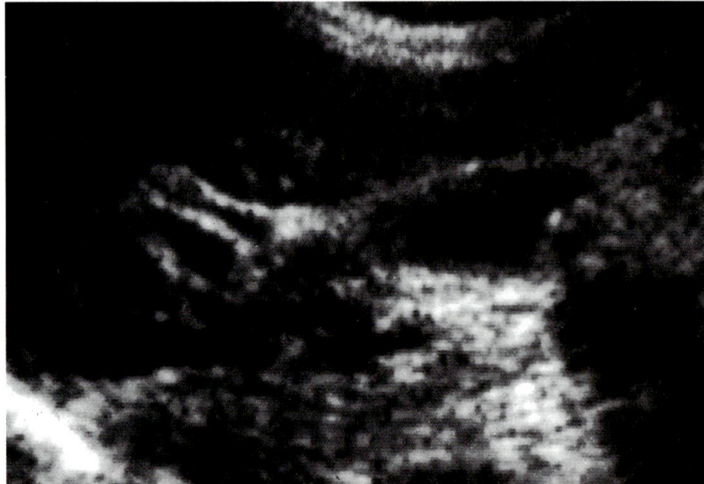

Fig. 6.1 Acute cholecystitis. Ultrasonography showing a dilated gall bladder containing sludge and a single gallstone, with pericholecystic effusion. By courtesy of Dr R. Noble.

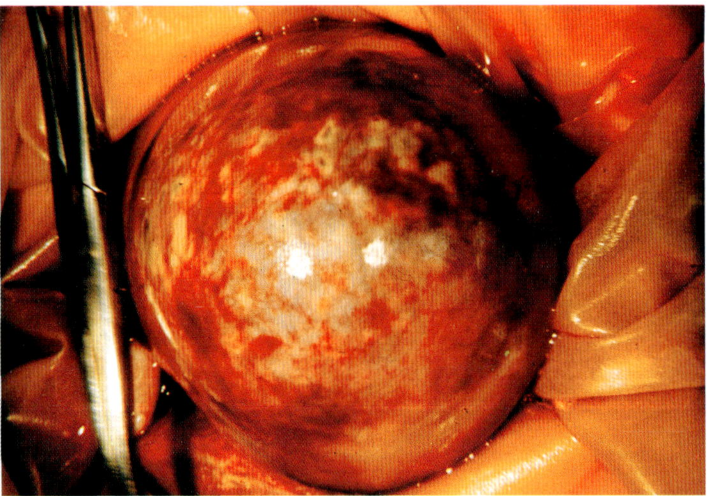

Fig. 6.2 Acute cholecystitis. Operating room photograph showing multiple dark greenish areas with surrounding yellow border on surface of gallbladder, indicating transmural necrosis. There is also marked vascular engorgement of the serosal surface, indicative of the severity of the inflammatory process, and greyish areas of exudate on the serosal surface. By courtesy of Dr M. Anderson.

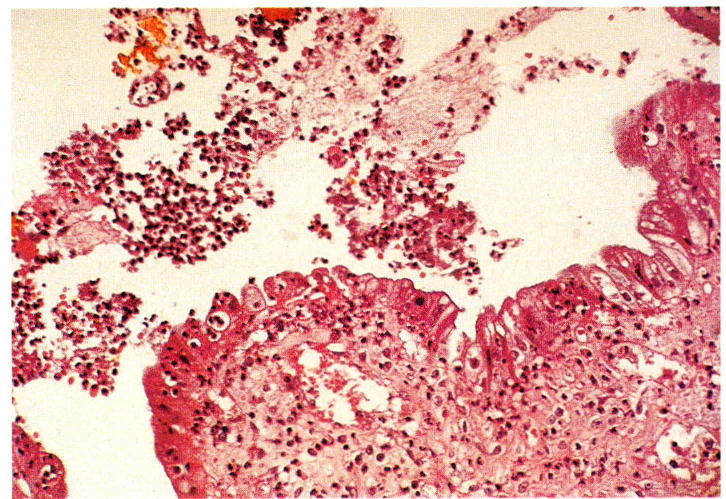

Fig. 6.3 Acute cholecystitis. Histological section of gallbladder mucosa and submucosa. Note the purulent exudate in the lumen and infiltration within the epithelial lining and mucosa. H&E stain. By courtesy of Professor M. S. R. Huth.

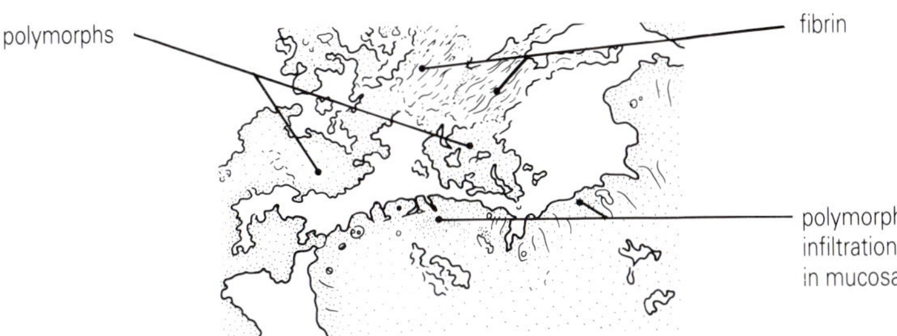

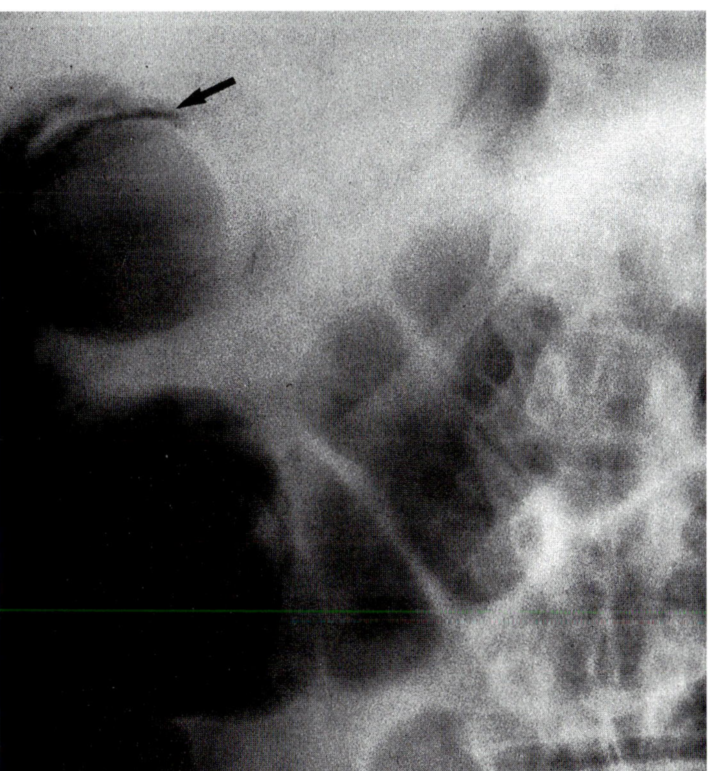

Fig. 6.4 Emphysematous cholecystitis: plain abdominal X-ray. The gallbladder is seen as a gas-filled viscus. Gas is present in the wall of the gallbladder due to infection by *Clostridium perfringens*. By courtesy of Dr M. Anderson.

stones may be present inside the gallbladder, and chronic inflammatory changes and fibrosis may be apparent in the wall and on the serosal surface (Fig. 6.5).

Most cases of acute cholecystitis resolve within a few days, but elderly or seriously ill patients, or those who develop complications such as perforation or gangrenous (emphysematous) cholecystitis, should be treated with antibiotics effective against gram-negative bacilli and anaerobic bacteria, e.g. piperacillin, mezlocillin, or a combination of an aminoglycoside plus metronidazole or clindamycin. Immediate surgical intervention (cholecystectomy or cholecystectomy with drainage) is required for perforation, pericholecystic abscess or gangrenous cholecystitis. Acute cholecystitis is often associated with extension of infection into the extrahepatic and intrahepatic biliary system (ascending cholangitis – Fig. 6.6). The cholangitis may become complicated by multiple intrahepatic abscesses (Fig. 6.7).

Ascending cholangitis usually produces severe systemic illness with high fever and chills, jaundice and severe pain and tenderness over the liver. Charcot's triad (fever, chills and jaundice) is present in 85% of cases. Ascending cholangitis is frequently associated with bacteraemia; the organisms isolated most commonly are *E. coli*, *Bacteroides*

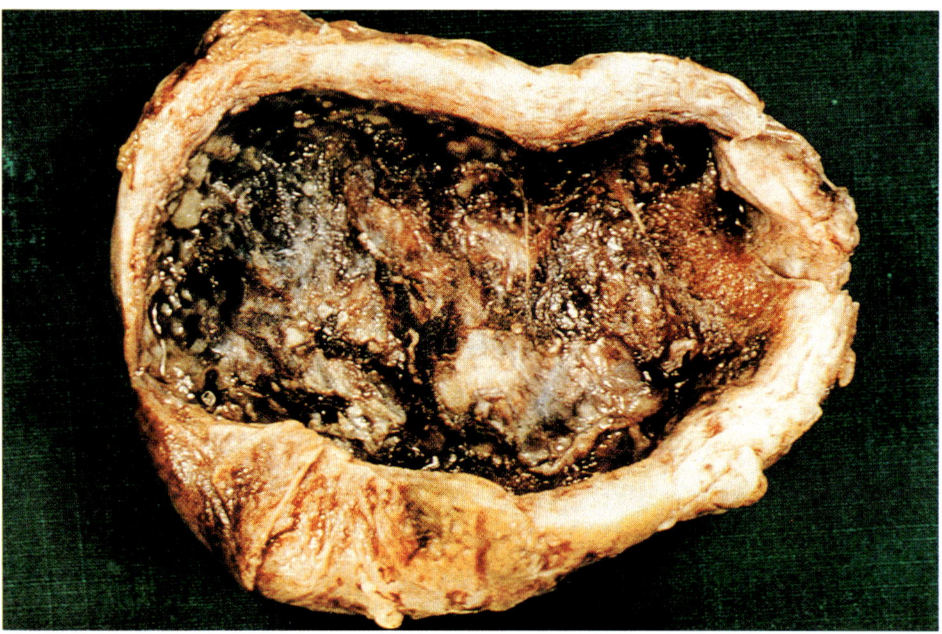

Fig. 6.5 Acute on chronic cholecystitis. Macroscopic specimen showing loss of mucosa and necrosis, with haemorrhage in the submucosa (acute changes). There is also marked thickening of the gallbladder wall secondary to scarring, multiple stones lining the lumen of the gallbladder, and a shaggy nontranslucent appearance to the serosal surface (chronic changes).

fragilis and *Clostridium perfringens.* Prompt therapy with appropriate antibiotics administered intravenously and relief of biliary obstruction is required. The technique of endoscopic retrograde cholangio-pancreatography (ERCP) has revolutionized the diagnosis and treatment of this condition

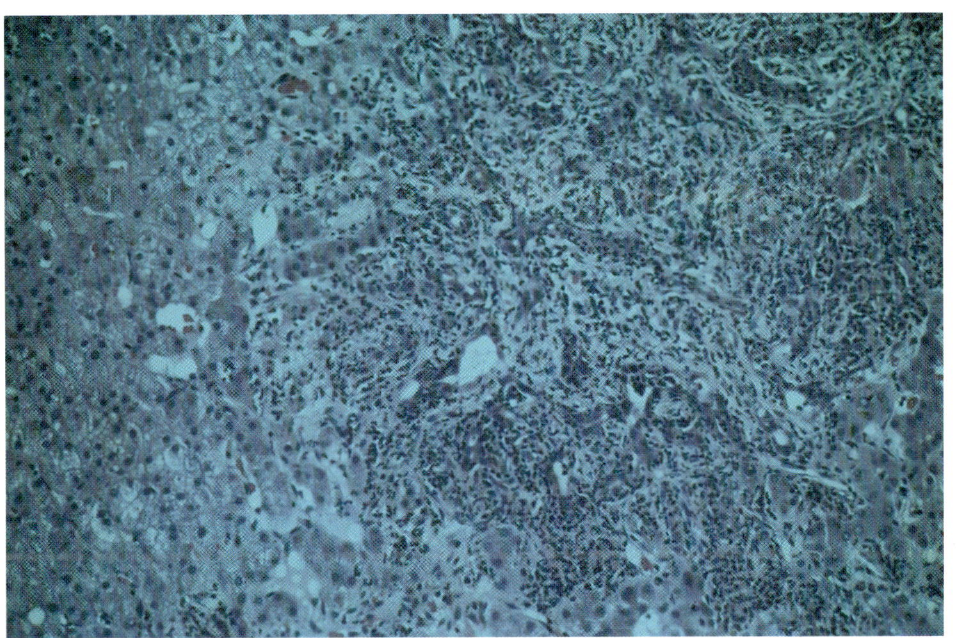

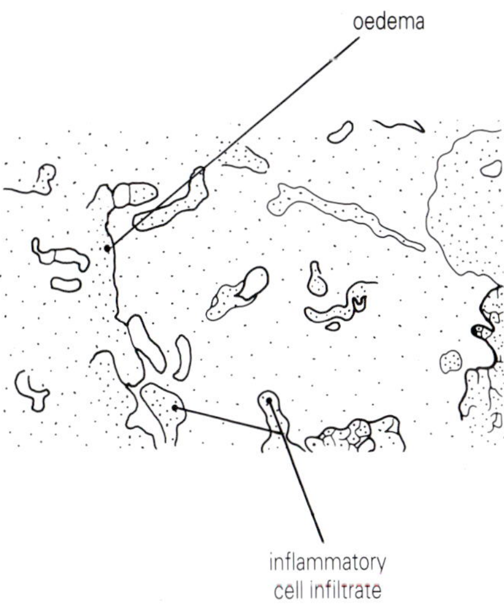

Fig. 6.6 Ascending cholangitis. The portal tract is oedematous and filled with inflammatory cells.

by allowing direct visualization of gallstones in the common bile duct (see Fig. 6.7). Either sphinctero-tomy with stone extraction (Fig. 6.8) or non-operative decompression of the biliary system by placement of an indwelling stent (Fig. 6.9) may be employed to relieve the obstruction.

CLONORCHIASIS

Man is an incidental host for the oriental liver fluke *Clonorchis sinensis*, a parasite of fish-eating mammals of the Far East. Millions of people in China and Southeast Asia are infected with this organism. The adult worms live in the distal biliary passages (Fig. 6.10), where they produce eggs which pass down the biliary system and out of the body in the faeces. The eggs are ingested by snails, in which they hatch into miracidia. These multiply within the snail, producing large numbers of cercariae that emerge into the water. The cercariae penetrate under the scales of certain freshwater fish, in which they encyst as metacercariae, the forms which are infective when ingested by mammals.

Man acquires the disease by eating inadequately cooked fish. The metacercariae encyst in the duodenum and pass through the ampulla of Vater, where they mature into adult worms inside the bile ducts. Most infected individuals are asymptomatic, but heavy infection may produce cholangitis and hepatitis. Infection with this fluke is associated with an increased incidence of adenocarcinoma arising from the epithelium of the bile ducts. Diagnosis is made by finding the characteristic eggs in the faeces. No satisfactory treatment for this infection is available.

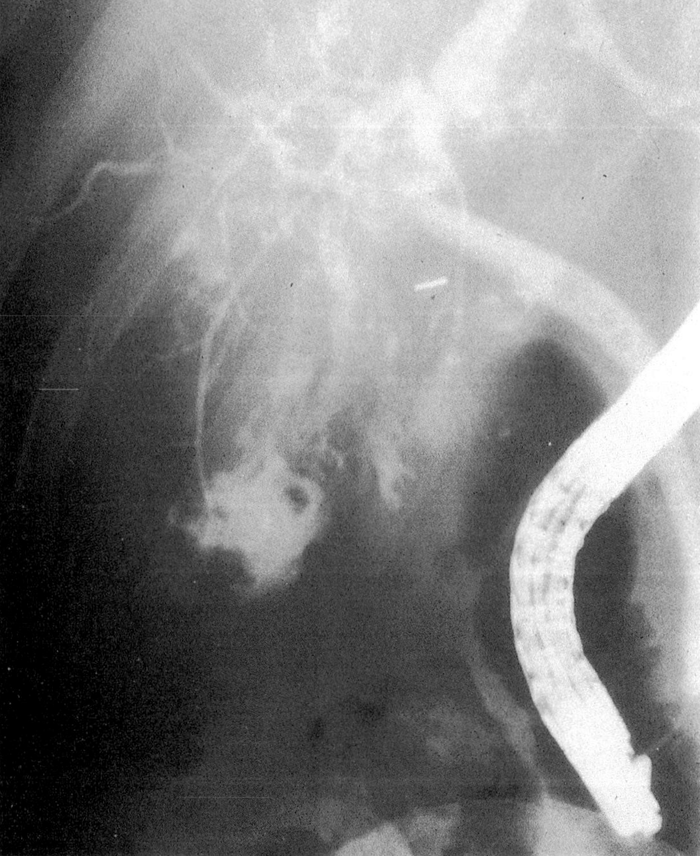

Fig. 6.7 Ascending cholangitis. Multiple intrahepatic abscesses and several stones in the common bile duct demonstrated by ERCP. The endoscope is visible in the lower right hand corner. By courtesy of Dr J. T. Cunningham.

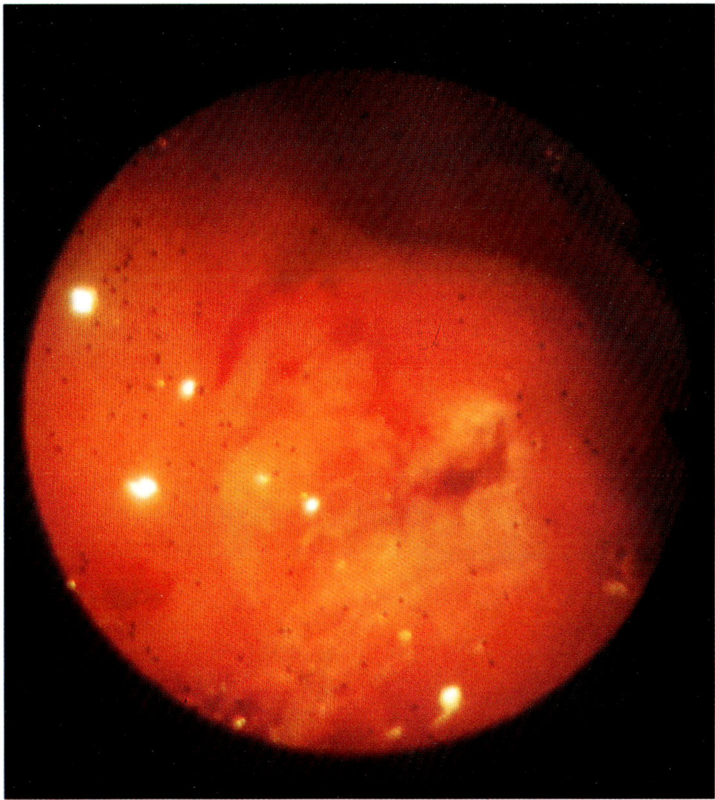

Fig. 6.8 Ascending cholangitis. Endoscopic view showing sphincterotomy of ampulla of Vater in treatment of ascending cholangitis. By courtesy of Dr J. T. Cunningham.

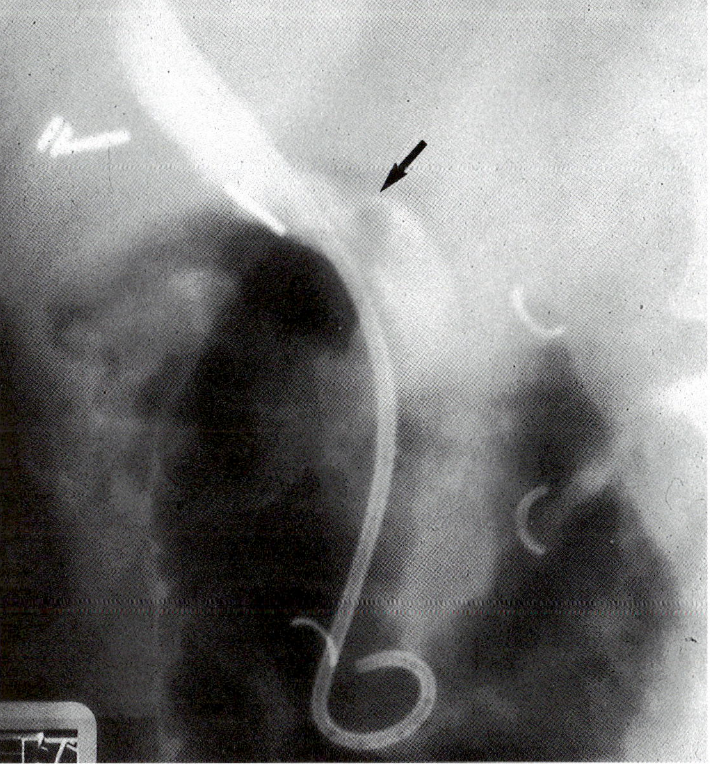

Fig. 6.9 Ascending cholangitis. A double pig-tailed endoprosthesis has been placed by ERCP to bypass the single stone in the common bile duct to prevent recurrent cholangitis. By courtesy of Dr J. T. Cunningham.

FASCIOLIASIS

Infection with the liver fluke *Fasciola hepatica* occurs throughout the world wherever sheep are raised. The adult worms live in the biliary system of sheep, cattle and man (Fig. 6.11), where they deposit their eggs. The eggs pass into the intestines and are eliminated in the faeces. They complete their development into miracidia in fresh water and infect the intermediate snail host. Multiplication occurs within the snail and cercariae emerge and undergo encystment into metacercariae attached to aquatic plants. When these are ingested they excyst and the larvae penetrate the intestinal wall and peritoneum, passing through the capsule of the liver and eventually reaching the biliary tract. The clinical illness is characterized by fever, eosinophilia and painful enlargement of the liver. Occasional cases have resulted in biliary obstruction or cirrhosis. Diagnosis is made by finding the eggs in faeces or bile. There is no proven effective treatment for the infection.

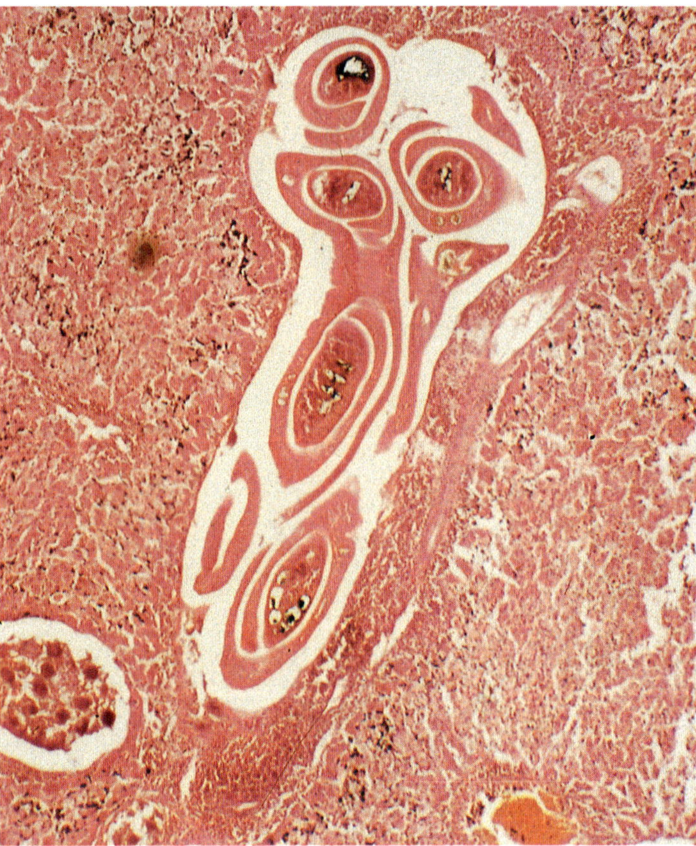

Fig. 6.10 Clonorchiasis. Section of liver showing multiple adult worms of *Clonorchis sinensis* in a distal biliary duct. H&E stain.

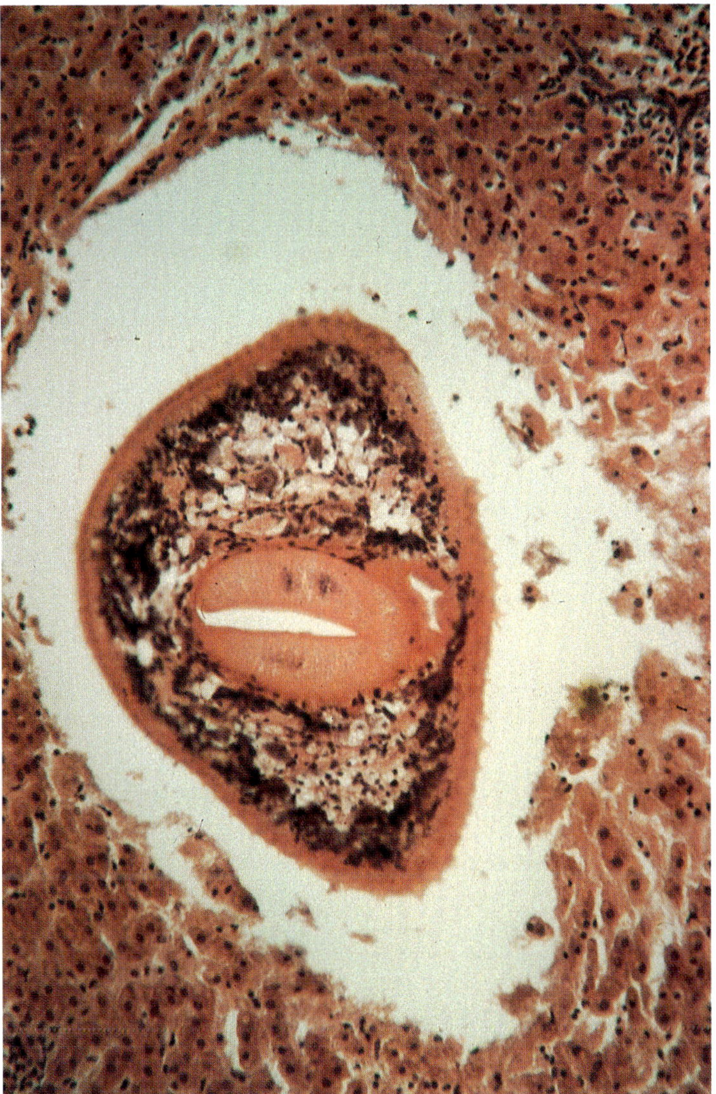

Fig. 6.11 Fascioliasis. Section of liver showing adult worm of *Fasciola hepatica* lying within a bile duct. H&E stain.

N

nalidixic acid 20, 23

Necator americanus 84–6

necrosis, hepatic 109, 110

necrotizing enteritis 35, 36

niclosamide 74, 76, 77

nitrofurans 8

non-A, non-B hepatitis virus 116–18

non-agglutinable (NAG) vibrios 15–16

Norwalk virus 92–3

nystatin 5

O

oesophagus

    infectious oesophagitis 2–6

    varices in chronic schistosomiasis 72, 128

P

paromomycin 68, 74, 76, 77

penicillin 51

penicillin G 35

Pepto-bismol 20

pericholecystic abscess 102

peritoneal dialysis 100, 103

peritonitis 100–103

    tuberculous 103, 104

pig-bel (necrotizing enteritis) 35, 36

pinworm 78

piperacillin 144

piperazine citrate 82

polyarteritis nodosa 114

polyarthritis 34

praziquantel 72, 74, 75, 76, 77, 138

probenecid 28

pseudo-appendicitis syndrome 31, 34

pseudomembranous colitis 22, 36–40

Pseudomonas aeruginosa liver abscess 134

pyrimethamine–sulphadoxine 66

Q

Q fever 122

quinacrine 65

quinolones 20

R

rectal spirochaetosis 41

Reye's syndrome 123–4, 125

rice water stool 14, 15

rifabutine 46

rifampin 28

rose spots 26, 27

rotaviruses 90–91

S

salmonella

    bacterial liver abscesses 133

    S. choleraesuis 28–9

    S. enteritidis 28–9

    S. typhi 23–8

salmonellosis 23–9

sarcoidosis 130

Schistosoma haematobium 28, 69–72

Schistosoma japonicum 69–72, 128

Schistosoma mansoni 69–72, 128, 129

schistosome dermatitis (swimmer's itch) 71

schistosomiasis 69–72, 73

    hepatic granulomas 128, 129

Sereny test 12

serum hepatitis (hepatitis B) 109–15

Shigella boydii 21

Shigella dysenteriae 20–21, 22

Shigella flexneri 21, 22

Shigella sonnei 21

shigellosis (dysentery) 11, 20–23

sphincterotomy 146, 147

spiramycin 65